EMERGENCIES in OBSTETRICS and GYNECOLOGY

CLINICS in EMERGENCY MEDICINE

VOL. 1

Forthcoming Volumes in the Series

Vol. 2 Resuscitation, Sheldon Jacobson, M.D., Guest Editor

Vol. 3 Controversies in Trauma Management, Robert H. Dailey, M.D., and Michael Callaham, M.D., Guest Editors

Vol. 4 The Intoxicated Patient, C. W. Hanson, M.D., Guest Editor

EMERGENCIES in OBSTETRICS and GYNECOLOGY

Edited by

Arnold W. Cohen, M.D.

Assistant Professor of Obstetrics and Gynecology
University of Pennsylvania School of Medicine
Philadelphia, Pennsylvania

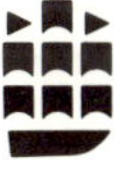

Churchill Livingstone
New York, Edinburgh, London, and Melbourne
1981

Distributed in the United Kingdom by Churchill Livingstone, Robert Stevenson House, 1-3 Baxter's Place, Leith Walk, Edinburgh EH1 3AF and by associated companies, branches and representatives throughout the world.

First published 1981

Printed in USA

ISBN 0-443-08130-1

7 6 5 4 3 2 1

Library of Congress Cataloging in Publication Data
Main entry under title:

Emergencies in obstetrics and gynecology.

(Clinics in emergency medicine; v. 1)
Includes bibliographies and index.
Contents: Obstetric and gynecological history and examination/Robert M. Liston—Drugs in pregnancy/Michael T. Mennuti—The acute abdomen in pregnancy/James R. Huey, Jr.—[etc.]
1. Pregnancy, Complications of. 2. Gynecologic emergencies. I. Cohen, Arnold W. II. Series. [DNLM: 1. Emergencies. 2. Genital diseases, Female. 3. Obstetrics. Wl CL831BCP v. 1/WP 100 C678e]
RG571.E46 618 81-12221
ISBN 0-443-08130-1 AACR2

Contributors

Arnold W. Cohen, M.D.
Assistant Professor of Obstetrics and Gynecology
University of Pennsylvania School of Medicine
Philadelphia, Pennsylvania

William R. Crombleholme, M.D., F.A.C.O.G.
Assistant Professor
Department of Obstetrics and Gynecology
Downstate Medical Center
Brooklyn, New York

Ralph T. DePalma, M.D.
Assistant Professor of Obstetrics and Gynecology
University of Texas
Southwestern Medical School at Dallas
Dallas, Texas

Gertrude J. Frishmuth, M.D.
Assistant Professor of Obstetrics and Gynecology
University of Pennsylvania School of Medicine
Assistant Surgeon
Department of Gynecology
Children's Hospital of Philadelphia
Philadelphia, Pennsylvania

Gilbert G. Haas, Jr., M.D.
Assistant Professor
Department of Obstetrics and Gynecology
Division of Human Reproduction
University of Pennsylvania School of Medicine
Philadelphia, Pennsylvania

James R. Huey, Jr., M.D.
Director of Obstetrics
St. Elizabeth Medical Center
Dayton, Ohio

Robert M. Liston, M.B., Ch.B, M.R.C.O.G.
Assistant Professor of Obstetrics and Gynecology
University of Pennsylvania School of Medicine
Philadelphia, Pennsylvania

Michael T. Mennuti, M.D.
Associate Professor of Obstetrics & Gynecology and Human Genetics
University of Pennsylvania School of Medicine
Philadelphia, Pennsylvania

Jan Schneider, M.D.
Professor and Chairman
Department of Obstetrics and Gynecology
Medical College of Pennsylvania
Philadelphia, Pennsylvania

Steven J. Sondheimer, M.D.
Assistant Professor
Department of Obstetrics and Gynecology
University of Pennsylvania School of Medicine
Philadelphia, Pennsylvania

Robert S. Weinstein, M.D.
Clinical Assistant Professor
Department of Obstetrics and Gynecology
University of Pennsylvania School of Medicine
Philadelphia, Pennsylvania

Preface

Every physician in a medical specialty will occasionally encounter emergency situations outside his or her own area of expertise. The Emergency Room physician, however, must routinely face problems of diagnosis and treatment covering a broad range of disciplines. This volume reviews the essential information required for the successful management of the gynecologic and obstetrical problems most often encountered in the Emergency Room. These problems may be as trivial as a diaphragm that cannot be extracted from the vagina or as life threatening as a hypotensive patient with an ectopic pregnancy. The authors of each chapter are practicing Obstetrician-Gynecologists in University settings who deal with these problems daily. They have expertise not only in the theoretical considerations of the specific problems, but in the practical management as well. Each chapter reviews the necessary anatomy and physiology before discussing specific management plans. Dosages of useful medications have been included in easily identifiable tables so that the chapters can be used as a quick reference guide for any physician dealing with the health care of women.

Dr. Robert Liston introduces the reader to the proper method of history taking and physical examination of the female patient. He stresses both the technique of a proper pelvic examination and the psychologic factors that must be considered if important historical data is to be obtained from the patient.

Any woman of reproductive age who presents to the Emergency Room may or may not be pregnant. Before any medication can be dispensed to the patient, the treating physician must be aware of what effect a specific drug has on the fetus. Dr. Michael Mennuti discusses the concepts of organogenesis and teratogenic agents before reviewing specific commonly prescribed medications.

Pregnant patients may suffer from any illness that occurs in the non-pregnant female, as well as those that specifically occur during the 282 days of gestation. Bleeding and pain during the first trimester may be so benign as to require only bed rest but they also may be the presenting symptoms for an acute intraabdominal emergency which, when not treated expeditiously by the emergency room physician, can result in a maternal mortality. Dr. Steven Sondheimer reviews these problems. Bleeding in the third trimester requires a cautious approach by the examining physician so that no further insult to the fetoplacental unit or mother will occur. Dr. William Crombleholme outlines a management plan and gives guidance for the follow-up treatment by the trained obstetrician. Drs. Huey, DePalma, and Cohen discuss medical complications during pregnancy which may require rapid treatment prior to any obstetrical intervention. The necessity of insuring the health of the mother and then the fetus is stressed in all of these chapters.

Abnormal hormonal interactions in the gynecologic patient usually present with irregular menses. Reassurance alone is adequate for many patients. However, the complex interaction of the hypothalmic-pituitary-ovarian-adrenal axes may have to be modified to adequately treat hypo- or hypermenorrhea as well as poly- or oligomenorrhea. Dr. Gil Haas describes the use of estrogenic, progestational, andogenic, and cortisol-like compounds to treat these women. The risk versus benefit of contraceptive modalities must be considered for the individual prior to therapy. Each effective contraceptive method is reviewed by Dr. Jan Schneider. The complications and management of those problems that may require treatment in the Emergency Room are delineated.

Vaginitis is probably the most common gynecologic complaint. Although often considered trivial by the treating physician, the physical and psychologic discomfort suffered by the patient can be monumental. Dr. Robert Weinstein reviews the common pathogens, predisposing factors, therapy, and follow-up necessary to adequately care for such problems.

Pediatric and adolescent gynecology, a field that has been neglected up until the late 1970's, is presented by Dr. Gertrude Frishmuth, who heads the pediatric gynecologic clinic at the Children's Hospital of Philadelphia. The genital tract of the prepubertal female is subject to different diseases than those seen after menarche. Furthermore, the new sexuality of the adolescent poses problems that were not even talked about 10 years ago.

I want to thank all the contributors for their excellent chapters and their promptness in meeting deadlines. A special thanks has to be given to Mrs. Michele Simons for her untiring efforts in typing and re-typing each chapter multiple times before the publisher received them. Marcia Cohen, my wife, also must be recognized not only for her support, but for her proof reading efforts as well. Through the work of these individuals, I believe a volume has been prepared which will serve as a guide to the understanding and treatment of the common gynecologic and obstretrical problems seen in the Emergency Room.

Arnold W. Cohen, M.D.

Contents

1. Obstetric and Gynecological History and Examination 1
Robert M. Liston

2. Drugs in Pregnancy 11
Michael T. Mennuti

3. The Acute Abdomen in Pregnancy 25
James R. Huey, Jr.

4. Hypertensive Disorders of Pregnancy 39
Ralph T. DePalma

5. Acute Medical Emergencies in Obstetrics 49
Arnold W. Cohen

6. Lower Abdominal Pain 61
Steven J. Sondheimer

7. Abnormal Vaginal Bleeding 81
Gilbert G. Haas, Jr.

8. Contraceptive Problems 103
Jan Schneider

9. Vaginitis 113
Robert S. Weinstein

10. Pediatric Gynecology 127
Gertrude J. Frishmuth

11. Bleeding During Pregnancy 135
William R. Crombleholme

Index 145

1 Obstetric and Gynecological History and Examination

Robert M. Liston

When face to face with the patient during the interview and examination, the two facets of the physician, artist and scientist, come closest together. The scientist demands that certain facts be ascertained, but it is only by intelligent inquiry, carefully worded and artfully presented, that this necessary information can be elicited. The most astute examiner is useless if his approach to the patient precludes a rapport and inhibits relaxation. Volumes have been written on the art of history taking and the method of physical examination. It is beyond the scope of this primer to be all embracing on the subject. The reader is referred to the standard works on physical examination and to sections in the classic textbooks of gynecology. The purpose of this chapter is to highlight certain aspects of the history and examination. This should be helpful to the emergency room physician in arriving at a correct diagnosis and thus initiating proper treatment with minimum delay. In an ideal world, the emergency room physician would encroach on the field of obstetrics and gynecology only in dealing with acute problems of early pregnancy, cases of trauma to the genital tract, and in the differential diagnosis of acute abdominal pain. However, in today's world, he may be called on, as is clear from later chapters in this volume, to advise about a missed period, to search for a lost tampon, or to handle many other common obstetric or gynecologic problems. The patient with any kind of complication of a pregnancy of more than 12 weeks gestation should probably be evaluated by the obstetric staff. Nevertheless, since such complications are often life threatening conditions that are readily amenable to therapy, mention is made of relevant points in the history and examination as an aid to prompt diagnosis and rapid referral to the obstetrician.

HISTORY

"The most important evidence is always provided by the history the patient or her relatives can give—if allowed to do so."—Sir Norman Jeffcoate

In obtaining a history, however brief, even in the bustle of the emergency room, an interested, sympathetic approach is vital. Apart from obtaining vital information which will often indicate the diagnosis, history taking provides an opportunity to build a relationship with the patient. This is necessary if she is going to allow herself to have a pelvic examination that provides the maximum amount of information. It is important to ascertain the patient's vital statistics: age, parity, previous obstetric history, previous medical and surgical history, menstrual pattern, date of the last menstrual period, sexual activity, and her mode, if any, of contraception. The above data base serves as a yardstick against which to measure her current complaint. Most patients in the emergency room with problems relating to the genital tract will complain of pain, bleeding, or both. Further inquiry into these two complaints is required and will be discussed. Finally a brief review of systems is important, even in the most seemingly obvious case, since it helps to exclude the presence of bowel or urinary tract pathology.

Data Base

The patient's age is a very important factor in the evaluation of any complaint referable to the female genital tract. In any patient between the ages of 15 and 50, the possibility of pregnancy should always be foremost in the physician's mind. The most important causes of uterine bleeding in women of such an age are associated with disorders of reproduction. In younger girls, bleeding is more likely to be due to an endocrine factor; in postmenopausal women, malignancy must be considered.

The patient's parity is also important. She may know that she is pregnant, and this may have been documented by a previous pelvic examination, pregnancy test, or ultrasonogram. She may have a history of recurrent abortions and know well the signs and symptoms of such an event. If so, a reaction to any

Table 1-1. History.

Data Base—age, parity, occupation, previous OB history, previous medical/surgical history, menstrual history and LMP, drug ingestion, sexual activity, contraception
Presenting Complaint:
Pain—location, onset and radiation, character, associated symptoms
Bleeding—altered menstruation, amenorrhea, intermenstrual, contact, drugs, associated symptoms
Discharge—onset and duration, color, consistency, odor, associated symptoms, pain, bleeding, pruritis

pain or bleeding may be colored by her past experience. Likewise, a history of infertility may give a clue to the diagnosis, especially if endometriosis or chronic pelvic infection has been documented in the past. A history of previous second or third trimester pregnancy loss should particularly alert the physician. A patient with an established pregnancy, complaining of pelvic pressure, lower abdominal pain, or leakage of fluid from the vagina, merits careful evaluation. Obviously, a past medical or surgical history may give important clues to the diagnosis. Of particular importance would be knowledge of a previous appendectomy, previous tubal or ovarian surgery, or a history of documented cardiovascular, respiratory, or bleeding disorder.

In any patient of reproductive age, menstrual history is extremely important. The age of onset of menstruation, the frequency and duration of periods, the character of the bleeding, and associated symptoms should all be ascertained. The date of the last normal menstrual period is a good starting point, but it is often easier, particularly when there is irregular and uncharacteristic vaginal bleeding, to record the timing of all such bleeding over the preceding several months. Since many patients will ascribe the name "period" to all vaginal bleeding, only by such an approach does it become clear what was menstrual and what was intermenstrual bleeding. It is only by ascertaining what is normal for any individual that one can determine the likely significance of an unusual bleeding pattern.

It is imperative to know if a given patient is sexually active, and if so, what, if any, contraception she is employing. However, we have all seen an ectopic pregnancy in a girl who has "never had intercourse." An unusual bleeding pattern may be explained by hormone preparations taken for contraception, but pregnancies can and do occur, although rarely, in patients who reliably take oral contraceptive medication. The presence of an intrauterine contraceptive device may be a basis for increased menstrual bleeding, intermenstrual bleeding, or uterine cramps. In addition, it may lead one to suspect pelvic infection or ectopic pregnancy.

Some of the particulars in this "data base" will be very obvious and many of the others can be ascertained very quickly, but its purpose is to paint a profile of the individual patient that serves as a ready reference point for her complaints to help in arriving at a rational diagnosis.

Pain

Many of the patients with gynecological emergencies will present with abdominal pain. It is important to remember that any female patient, pregnant or otherwise, is capable of having pain due to pathology arising anywhere in the abdomen and not solely from the genital tract. However, certain features of pain may make the latter a more distinct possibility. The site and radiation of the pain is an important clue in arriving at a diagnosis. Pain of uterine origin tends to be felt diffusely over the hypogastrium. It is often referred to the inner aspects of the thighs. Adnexal pain is usually felt lower in the abdomen, in the area just above the inguinal ligament. Abdominal pain may be accompanied with backache, or the latter may occur by itself. Backache of pelvic origin tends to be felt in the midline and usually occurs over the sacrum. Throbbing pain in the midline is typical of abortion, but it may be preceded by general lower pelvic ache and discomfort for several days. An early tubal abortion may also give rise to cramp-like pains, but usually the pain is felt more to one side or the other. A lancinating pain of sudden onset may be appreciated with an acute tubal rupture. In this situation the rest of the history and examination will usually make the diagnosis. The pain of pelvic inflammatory disease is usually appreciated as a constant dull ache. It is classically bilateral, although it may be initially felt on one side only. Again, rupture of a tubal abscess may give rise to severe, piercing lower abdominal pain with the rapid development of diffuse abdominal discomfort. Irritation of the diaphragm by intraabdominal fluid or blood may give rise to referred shoulder tip pain. This occurs in about 10 percent of cases of ruptured ectopic pregnancy. Pain due to torsion of an ovarian cyst may initially be localized low in the iliac fossa, but it may become more generalized as the process progresses. Torsion is often associated with nausea, vomiting, and a slight pyrexia. The occurrence of a right sided cyst may be mistaken for an acute appendicitis. Often, however, there is a history of intermittent preceding bouts of dull pain or even occasional attacks of sharp, localized pain. It is clear then that related features may help in the differential diagnosis of pain. Such features should be carefully elicited in the history. The patient may know she is pregnant and the gestational age of the pregnancy may indicate the cause of the pain. If the pregnancy is advanced beyond 12 weeks, midline pain might suggest an impending abortion, and such pain occurring beyond 20 weeks might suggest premature labor or placental abruption. In either case, prompt attention by the obstetrician is imperative.

The relationship of the pain to menstruation or other bleeding is also helpful in forming a diagnosis. Very often pain of pelvic inflammatory disease begins at the end of menstruation. Although bleeding and pain may present together in a case of abortion, it is more common for the bleeding to precede and overshadow the pain in the initial stages. With a tubal abortion, however, pain is often appreciated before vaginal bleeding occurs. Indeed, a history of dull unilateral cramp-like pain, occurring for several days or even weeks prior to the patient presenting, may be obtained.

The presence of a vaginal discharge might be helpful in forming a diagnosis. The physician should always question the patient about this. Chronic pelvic inflammatory disease may not be associated with any increase in vaginal discharge, but it is usually present in cases of acute salpingitis. Lower abdominal pain and pelvic discomfort due to chronic cervicitis or severe vaginitis might be revealed by an increase in vaginal discharge. Although vaginitis and its associated discharge are common in early pregnancy, it is unusual to find active salpingitis and pregnancy co-existing. The presence of a purulent discharge from the cervical os would make the diagnosis of a pregnancy complication extremely unlikely.

The degree of systemic upset and its relationship to the pain should be ascertained. Symptoms of pregnancy may predominate and suggest the diagnosis of a pregnancy complication. Thus the presence or absence of nausea, vomiting, breast tenderness, and fatigue should be ascertained. Fever and nausea are usually found in cases of salpingitis, but vomiting itself occurs only in severe cases. Vomiting may occur with torsion of an ovarian cyst, but generally speaking it is unusual in gynecological emergencies. As mentioned in the introduction, an inquiry into urinary and bowel symptoms may help in differentiating the different causes of pain.

Bleeding

As has been previously mentioned, no history of bleeding can properly be evaluated without detailed knowledge of the patient's normal menstrual cycle. Only with this standard for a reference can one begin to interpret a complaint of abnormal bleeding. Any change in the interval, duration, or amount of menstrual bleeding is important. Classically, a history of amenorrhea followed by bleeding raises the question of some accident of early pregnancy, but often, particularly in cases of ectopic pregnancy, amenorrhea may be absent. In a case of tubal abortion, bleeding usually continues once it starts, but it is seldom copious in amount. During a miscarriage, bleeding is intermittent. It can be accompanied with the passage of clots. As noted above, the relationship of the bleeding with any associated pain is important to ascertain. Because of the absence of amenorrhea from the history in many cases of tubal pregnancy, the mistaken diagnosis of intermenstrual bleeding due to hormonal causes may be made. Intermenstrual bleeding may occur regularly, particularly in the younger patient. It may be associated with the use of an intrauterine contraceptive device or hormonal contraception. It must also be distinguished from contact bleeding, often precipitated by intercourse and occurring in cases of cervical erosion or polyp. Bleeding may also occur as a result of trauma, and any suggestion of this needs to be followed up by a further history. If it is clear from the history that the patient is 20 weeks or more in pregnancy, bleeding must be assumed to be due to premature cervical dilation, abruption, or placenta previa. In this situation, obstetric consultation should be obtained rapidly. Sometimes it is not clear to the patient that prescribed medications contain exogenous steroids which could be responsible for bleeding. In all cases of bleeding where the cause is not initially obvious, careful inquiry as to the use of drugs should be made.

Discharge

In any patient presenting with vaginal discharge, the physician should ascertain the duration and quantity of discharge. Some idea of its consistency, appearance, and odor should be obtained. The presence or absence of any associated pain or pruritis should also be recorded. Once again, such related symptoms as systemic upset, and urinary and bowel symptoms should be determined. By such inquiry, an indication as to the site and degree of any infection may be obtained. A discreet inquiry about the use of tampons or other "vaginal inserts" may be indicated. Once again, the patient who is pregnant presents a specific problem and the possibility of amniotic fluid leakage should always be kept in mind. After 14 weeks gestation, and certainly after 20 weeks gestation, such a question is best resolved by the obstetric service.

Trauma

In the patient presenting with a history of trauma to the genital area, attention to complaints of bleeding and pain are important. It is also obviously necessary to inquire about bladder function. Young girls, in whom it is difficult to visualize the vagina, or anybody in whom there is a question of a penetrating injury, even with a lack of symptoms on direct inquiry, should be referred for specialist evaluation.

EXAMINATION

General

Very often the diagnosis in a patient presenting to the emergency room with a gynecological complaint will be indicated by the history. Nevertheless, it is important that a full physical examination by carried out in order that a potentially dangerous misdiagnosis is not made. Of course, vital signs—temperature, pulse rate, blood pressure, respiratory rate—should be recorded on all patients. A brief general examination is then made. Examination of the breasts may reveal characteristic changes of pregnancy and may prompt a more searching abdominal and pelvic examination than might have been indicated by the patient's history. Inspection of the abdomen for mobility is helpful in the diagnosis of disseminated peritoneal irritation. This should be followed up by examination for tenderness, guarding, and rebound tenderness. The presence or absence of bowel signs should be noted and any mass carefully delineated. An operative scar on the abdomen may prompt further questioning of some historical point overlooked by the patient in the excitement of the moment. The mass most likely to be palpated in the emergency room setting is the uterus itself. It is well to remember that generally it is not palpable above the symphysis until 12 weeks of pregnancy have elapsed; in cases of retroversion, it may not be palpable until after 16 weeks. The absence of a palpable uterus does not exclude the diagnosis of a pregnancy complication. In cases of abortion, the uterus is often tender, and that tenderness is usually in the midline. This contrasts with cases of ectopic pregnancy, where the tenderness is more often unilateral, at least in the early stages, and may be associated with some guarding. Rebound tenderness is found where there has been leakage of blood from the tube, rupture of an ovarian cyst, or leakage from a tubo-ovarian abscess. Rigidity may be seen when such leakage is anything more than minimal. In cases of acute pelvic inflammation, tenderness, like the pain, is usually bilateral. With torsion of an ovarian cyst there may be acute, localized tenderness deep in the iliac fossa on the affected side, with overlying guarding. The area of tenderness becomes more diffuse as the process continues and gradually rigidity of the lower abdomen will ensue.

Pelvic Examination

The pelvic examination in many cases will serve to confirm a diagnosis suspected from the history and general examination. Because of the opportunity it affords to examine "hidden organs," it occasionally brings to light a previously unsuspected problem. No pelvic examination is easy either for the examiner or the patient, but, with the correct approach to each individual patient, one can develop a rapport and relaxed attitude so that the optimum benefit from such an examination can be achieved. The first essential in any pelvic examination is the consent of the patient. The examination should be conducted in private. If possible, a closed room should be used; this affords more security to the patient than a flimsy screen. All efforts to relax the patient are worthwhile, since without relaxation, the pelvic examination may be worse than useless. The presence of a third party is essential; preferably, this should be a female nurse or relative. A good nurse can accomplish much in helping the patient relax. Another essential is a good light for visualization of the vagina and the cervix. The complete pelvic examination should involve both inspection and palpation. It is useful to evolve a systematic approach. If the various organs (the vulva, vagina, cervix, body of uterus, appendages, and pouch of Douglas) are treated systematically, then omissions will not be made.

Inspection of the vulva might indicate trauma or the changes associated with vulvitis. In addition, there may be matted blood over the vulva or swelling of Bartholin's glands. Occasionally in the older patient, the cause of bleeding will be a vulvar lesion. Inspection of the vagina carried out by means of a bivalve speculum should always precede palpation. A note should be made of the presence or absence of any discharge or blood in the vagina. If blood is present, it should be collected and its volume ascertained. The appearance of any discharge should be carefully recorded. The white streaky adherent discharge of candidiasis should be contrasted with the creamy, frothy discharge seen in association with trichomonads. The source of the discharge should be elucidated: whether it comes directly from the vagina or from the cervix.

Table 1-2. Pelvic examination.

Inspection:
Vulva—blood, excoriation, inflammation, trauma
Vagina—inflammation, trauma, contents (blood, discharge, F.B.'s)
Cervix—appearance, discharge, bleeding
Palpation:
Cervical excitation
Cervical dilatation
Uterine size, consistency, tenderness
Adnexal tenderness, enlargement
Pouch of Douglas fullness, mass
Rectovaginal septum fixation, mass
Rectal mass, bleeding

Likewise, the source of any bleeding should be identified. Is bleeding coming from the vagina, from a local bleeding point caused by trauma, or is the blood exuding through the external os? The appearance of the cervix should then be studied. Does it look open? Is it well epithelialized, everted, eroded, or infected? A visual search for foreign bodies should be carried out, remembering that these, if lost, tend to reside in the posterior fornix and are often not appreciated until bimanual examination is carried out.

For internal examination, to palpate the pelvic organs, modern teaching favors the use of the right hand. One finger should be gently inserted in the posterior aspect of the vagina with pressure downwards on the perineal body. A second finger is then introduced along the posterior wall of the vagina. The hand is supinated to palpate the cervix. A positive effort should be made to determine the size, shape, position, mobility, and tenderness of the various organs. Remember that the Fallopian tubes are almost never palpable and the ovaries are often extremely difficult to palpate. Even an experienced examiner may record an absence of enlargement of the ovaries rather than the actual size of the ovaries themselves. In an emergency, it is useful, before bimanual palpation, simply to manipulate gently the cervix with the vaginal fingers. It is important to differentiate between the normal discomfort experienced by the patient during this procedure and pathologic pain. Pain suggests an inflammatory process or peritoneal irritation. The patency of the external os should be evaluated. A widely open soft cervix may indicate an inevitable or incomplete abortion.

From palpation of the cervix, one can proceed to palpation of the body of the uterus. Remember that in order to do this, the fingers in the vagina must be placed in the posterior fornix and the uterus elevated in the pelvis towards the abdominal wall anteriorly. With the flat of the abdominal hand, the uterus can be appreciated between the fingers of both hands. An approximation of the size and consistency of the uterus may then be obtained. The enlargement of a pregnant uterus is uniform and is accompanied by a degree of softening of the uterus. Enlargement of the uterus due to fibroids is irregular and imparts a firmness to the uterus. Tenderness of the uterus is usually due to infection, but it may also be found with threatened abortions. In chronic pelvic infection, the uterus may be immobile and it may feel large due to adhesion of bowel or ommentum.

After the uterus has been appreciated, attention is paid to the adnexa. If the patient has been complaining of unilateral pain, the painful side should be examined last. By careful bimanual examination, the presence or absence of any mass, and possibly its size and consistency, can be ascertained. In the emergency situation, however, usually an appreciation of tenderness is a more important diagnostic tool. In cases of ectopic pregnancy, it is very common for no mass to be appreciated, but acute tenderness on the affected side is usual. In acute salpingitis, tenderness is usually bilateral, and once again no masses are appreciated. An ovarian cyst may be felt, but if there is much pain and abdominal guarding, it may be difficult to delineate this fully. Once again only an impression of tenderness may be obtained.

Finally, attention should be paid to the pouch of Douglas. Fullness may be appreciated in cases where there has been bleeding into the pelvis. Occasionally an ovarian mass may be felt down behind the uterus. An organized pelvic hematocele may present a doughy appearance on palpation and may not be tender. Every pelvic examination should be concluded with a vaginorectal exam so that the rectal-vaginal septum can be palpated. This will also help to localize rectal pathology.

Special Cases

Although the keen emergency room physician will be eager to formulate a diagnosis by completing the examination on any obstetrical or gynecological emergency, there are certain patients in whom examination is contraindicated. Patients over 20 weeks pregnant with bleeding should certainly not be examined vaginally. Any patient over 12 weeks pregnant who has a story suggestive of leakage of amniotic fluid is probably best assessed by the obstetric consultant. Vaginal examination is usually difficult or impossible in a virgin. One may have to make an initial assessment with a rectal examination. Consideration of examination under anesthesia by the specialist may be necessary. Cases of trauma where there is a suggestion of a penetrating injury should, as already mentioned, be referred for specialist care and further examination. This is particularly true in any young girl where, if a vaginal examination is deemed necessary, it is best performed under some kind of anesthesia. In patients who claim to have been raped, or where there is a suspicion of rape, examination should be done by someone experienced in dealing with such allegations.

SUGGESTED READINGS

Cavanagh D, Woods RE, O'Connor TCF: Obstetric Emergencies. Harper & Row, Hagerstown, 1978.

Danforth NE: Obstetrics and Gynecology. Harper and Row, Hagerstown, 1977.

Jeffcoate Sir N: Principles of Gynaecology. Butterworths, London, 1975.

Kistner RW: Gynecology, Principles and Practice. Year Book Medical Publishers, Chicago, 1971.

MacLeod JG: Clinical Examination. Churchill Livingstone, Edinburgh, 1976.

Prior JA, Silverstein JS: Physical Diagnosis. C.V. Mosby, Saint Louis, 1973.

2 Drugs in Pregnancy

Michael T. Mennuti

Drugs administered to the pregnant patient may have profound effects on the fetus or neonate. These may range from fetal death followed by early abortion, to transient pharmacologic effects during the neonatal period. With the exception of obstetricians, physicians in emergency medicine probably have the most frequent occasion to prescribe medication for the pregnant patient. This most often occurs during early pregnancy; at times, even prior to the diagnosis of pregnancy. In many instances these medications are given for the relief of pregnancy related symptoms. Reassurance regarding the benign nature of these symptoms is sufficient for many patients rather than pharmacologic treatment. On the other hand, a medical complication requiring drug therapy presents a dilemma in establishing a risk/benefit ratio for both the mother and the fetus.

Media warnings designed to educate women to avoid unnecessary drug exposure have resulted in pregnant patients questioning the safety of prescribed medication, and have also caused them to have concern about medication taken at an earlier time during pregnancy. Difficulty in answering patient's questions regarding the safety of a drug often leads to a reluctance to prescribe medication for pregnant women even when there is a reasonable indication to do so. When considering a previous exposure, advice based solely on isolated case reports of humans with birth defects following use of an agent, or results of animal studies, may unjustifiably increase the patient's anxiety and, at times, lead to elective termination of wanted pregnancies. When followed by the birth of a child with an unrelated malformation, such counselling may serve to exaggerate maternal guilt feelings or anger toward the physician. It is the purpose of this chapter to review the potential effects of drugs on the fetus, and to consider how the available data might be used when treating or advising pregnant patients. Agents in current clinical use which have known or suspected teratogenic effects are described.

MAGNITUDE OF THE PROBLEM

In spite of the thalidomide disaster, studies of women in the United States since the 1950's indicate an increasing frequency of drug exposure during pregnancy. In a recent study, it was found that 93.4 percent of patients used 5 or more drugs during the prenatal period and the average number of drugs was 11.[1] Drugs used for pregnancy related symptoms,—analgesics, antihistamines, antinauseants, diuretics, laxatives—constitute a large proportion of the medications taken. It is possible that physician and patient awareness of this problem in the last few years has resulted in a reduction in the frequency of drug use during pregnancy, although this has not been documented.

This high frequency of drug use in our society raises legitimate concerns regarding the contribution of these agents to the occurrence of reproductive failure or birth defects. A major congenital malformation has been defined as any structural, functional, or biochemical abnormality in development, originating prior to birth or shortly thereafter, that causes immediate or delayed abnormality in structure or function of any organ. Major malformations occur in approximately 2 to 3 percent of all newborns.[2] Those malformations due to a definable etiology can be grouped according to whether they have a hereditary basis, or are thought to be due to environmental causes. Notably a substantial proportion of malformations remains unexplained. It has been estimated that perhaps only 2 percent of the malformations which occur in liveborns are attributable to a drug.[3] It is important, however, to recognize that genetic and environmental causes of malformations need not act as a single agent nor are they mutually exclusive. Because of the high frequency of drug use and the large proportion of malformations which remains unexplained, the possibility of drug-gene or drug-drug interaction should not be overlooked as potentially important in some cases.

PROBLEMS IN DEFINING HUMAN TERATOGENS

Three types of data are commonly available to evaluate the effects of drugs on fetal development: animal experiments, epidemiologic studies, and case reports. Each of these methods may have certain inherent limitations which can cause considerable difficulty in applying the information gained from them to the management of a patient.

Animal models are of primary value in studying the mechanisms of action of teratogens and may serve as a warning of potential teratogenic effects in humans. Nevertheless, caution must be exercised in extrapolating animal data directly to humans. Variation may occur in absorption, metabolism, drug distribution, protein binding, placental transfer, and genetic susceptibility between a particular animal strain and the human. For example, thalidomide, the most potent human teratogen, does not have similar effects in the rat, probably because the principle teratogenic metabolite is not formed in this species. A large proportion of drugs are teratogenic in laboratory animals using specific testing conditions. For many of these compounds there is no evidence to support a causal relationship between the drug and birth defects in humans. In spite of these limitations, it is reasonable, at times, to select alternative agents to a drug known to be an animal teratogen. This is particularly true for a newly marketed drug, if the metabolism and placental transfer are similar to that observed in humans, or if the established mechanism for teratogenicity in animals might also apply to the human situation.

Epidemiologic studies are particularly useful for identifying drugs which have a low level of teratogenicity. These agents, frequently referred to as *soft teratogens,* cause characteristic defects only in a small proportion of exposed pregnancies. It is important to recognize that an association of birth defects with use of a particular agent; e.g., a 1 to 2 fold increase, established by a retrospective study, may not imply a causal relationship. In such studies, bias of ascertainment is a frequent problem in that women who deliver an infant with a malformation are more likely to recall drug exposures during pregnancy than those who deliver a normal child. A confounding bias arises when there is an association of defects with the maternal disease or symptom being treated rather than the drug used. It is quite easy to understand how an association of insulin and congenital heart defects could be made, since these are among the most common malformations which are increased in frequency in infants of diabetic mothers. The occurrence of these defects is thought to be due to the maternal disease rather than the therapeutic agent. When reviewing an epidemiologic study associating a drug with malformations, it is reasonable to question if use of the drug might be frequently accompanied by use of another agent that may either interact with it, or of itself produce the teratogenic effect. For example, it is not unreasonable to expect that women who use minor tranquilizers might also more frequently abuse such social drugs as caffeine, tobacco, or alcohol. In spite of the problems in establishing a causal relationship from epidemiologic studies, empirically determined risks of these associations are at times useful for counselling patients or in establishing a risk/benefit ratio for treatment.

With the known population frequency of malformation it is not unexpected that case reports will be published of an infant with a defect following exposure to a drug. One would expect that the malformations which occur most frequently would predominate in these reports. Quite commonly, however, the tendency is to report very rare defects, complex defects, or those which have a causal relationship with a different agent (e.g., limb reduction due to thalidomide). This type of report frequently prompts reports of similar occurrences, resulting in the potentially fallacious assumption that the drug causes the particular defect. At times, reports of malformations which coincide embryologically with the gestational age of exposure to the drug, or are potentially a consequence of a known effect of a drug, raise even greater concern. In these instances, a causal relationship may be suspected, but because the denominator of the equation (i.e., number of specific defects per exposed pregnancy) is missing, the level of risk cannot be defined. A suspicion of teratogenicity raised by this type of report must be evaluated by carefully conducted prospective studies.

The criteria proposed for establishing a new drug as a potent human teratogen are: (1) an abrupt increase in the frequency of a particular defect or association of defects (syndrome); (2) coincidence of this increase with a known environmental change (e.g., widespread use of a new drug); (3) known exposure to the environmental change early in pregnancies yielding characteristically defective infants; and (4) absence of other factors common to the pregnancies yielding characteristically defective infants.

As expected, the number of agents which have met these criteria are relatively few. Nevertheless, because of the high frequency of drug use in our pregnant population, continuing surveillance for new teratogens, by each of the methods described, is extremely important.

FACTORS INFLUENCING THE TERATOGENIC POTENTIAL OF DRUGS

A variety of factors determines the teratogenic potential of a drug. The ability of the drug to cross the placenta is of primary importance. Mechanisms for placental transfer include: simple diffusion, facilitated diffusion, active transport, bulk flow, and pinocytosis. Simple diffusion, the most important mechanism for transfer of drugs, is dependent upon the concentration gradient between the maternal and fetal circulation. In addition, low molecular weight (less than 700 mw), high lipid solubility, low ionic charge, and low protein binding favor placental transfer. Relatively little information is available regarding production of differing drug metabolites during pregnancy or on an individual genetic basis. Notably, a drug metabolite may have greater or lesser potential for placental transfer and differing embryotoxic effects from the parent compound. Thus, unless there is sufficient human data to the contrary, it must be considered that a drug, or one of its metabolites, may cross the placenta by one or another mechanism and gain access to the fetus. The genetic constitution of the fetus (i.e., the liability for a particular defect) is probably the most important factor which accounts for the observation that teratogens may have variable effects in different species and most usually do not have adverse effects on all exposed human pregnancies. At the present time there is not sufficient information available to identify subgroups of patients who may be susceptible to embryotoxic effects of particular agents.

From a clinical point of view, the potential risks for the fetus are most readily assessed in terms of the gestational age at the time of exposure. Critical periods for exposure have been defined for several potent teratogens. These are generally limited to the time during embryonic development when organogenesis takes place (Fig. 2.1). Defects occurring during gametogenesis might result in reduced fertility, due to impairment of spermatogenesis or ovulation, gene mutation, or chromosomal errors. A causal relationship between

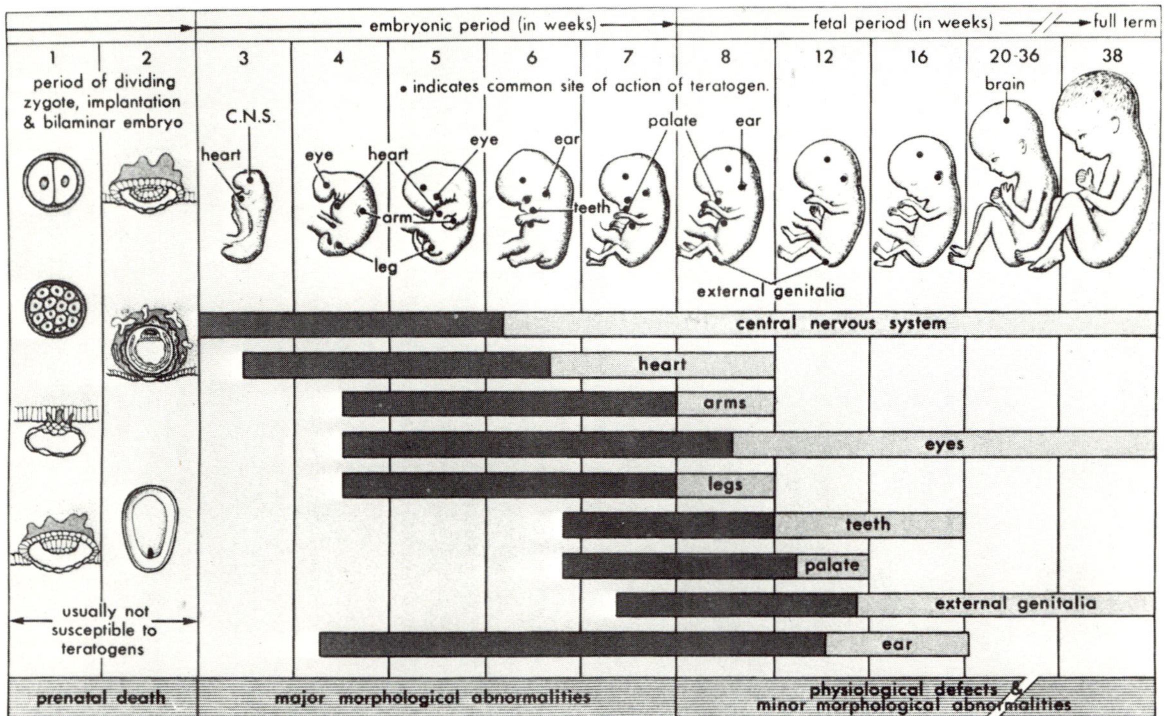

Fig. 2-1 Schematic illustration of the sensitive or critical periods in human development. Darkly shaded bar denotes highly sensitive periods; lightly shaded bar indicates stages that are less sensitive to teratogens. (Adapted from *The Developing Human: Clinically Oriented Embryology*, Keith L. Moore, W. B. Saunders Company, 1974, p. 117. Reproduced with the kind permission of the W. B. Saunders Company.)

drugs and new mutation or chromosome abnormalities has not been well established in humans. Preconceptual therapy with potentially toxic agents, for example cancer chemotherapy, is a frequent source of concern for patients and physicians. Studies in females receiving prior chemotherapy for malignancy have not demonstrated an adverse effect on future offspring.[4] Comparable studies have not been conducted in males. Because spermatogenesis takes place over a relatively short period of time (64 days) it is generally believed that prior drug therapy has no influence beyond this limited period of time.

For a number of years, reports of an increased number of chromosome breaks related to LSD caused speculation regarding the potential effect of this social drug on reproduction. Subsequent studies, however, have not established a relationship between this drug and chromosome abnormalities or malformations in the offspring. The possible effects of drugs used to induce ovulation, specifically clomiphene citrate, have also been considered. Case reports of malformed infants following ovulation induction may in fact only reflect a bias of reporting such occurrences. In a number of these cases, the infants have had neural-tube defects. It is not clear whether there is an increased frequency of these defects among offspring of women treated with these drugs, or if there might be an association of these defects with subfertility. The latter has been suggested by epidemiologic studies of the neural tube defects. One study has shown an increased frequency of Trisomy 21 infants born to women following induced ovulation.[5] This important observation should be further investigated because patients at increased risk for having a child with this disorder may wish to consider early prenatal cytogenetic diagnosis by amniocentesis.

The possibility of male mediated teratogenesis has been raised by case reports of thalidomide embryopathy following paternal, but not maternal, use of this drug, and a reported increased frequency of birth defects among children born of epileptic fathers. The detection of certain drugs (for example, hydantoin) in semen has fostered further speculation about this possibility. At present, paternal transmission of drugs is of great interest to teratologists, but is as yet unproven as being clinically important.

The first 2 weeks of early embryonic development (to menstrual age 4 weeks) appears to be both by clinical observations and animal experimentation, relatively insensitive to teratogenic effects. It seems likely that if there is an embryotoxic effect during this time, it would result in embryonic death and spontaneous abortion. Approximately 10 to 20 percent of recognized human conceptions terminate in early miscarriage. Of first trimester spontaneous abortions, about one-half are due to chromosome abnormalities. Other than a small fraction attributable to such factors as uterine abnormalities and maternal hormonal disorders, the remainder are unexplained. A recent association of increased maternal alcohol consumption with spontaneous abortions strongly suggests that there may be a causal relationship between this agent and pregnancy loss.[6,7] Associations between abortion and such other social drugs as tobacco and caffeine have been suggested, but the chromosomes of the pregnancies were not analyzed in these studies. An increased risk of abortion associated with chronic exposure to low concentrations of anesthetic gases in operating room personnel has been demonstrated by several large retrospective studies.[8] Recently a prospective study of this problem did not confirm this finding.[9] Because of the large number of unexplained spontaneous abortions, further studies of environmental factors or drugs common to pregnancies resulting in chromosomally normal abortuses should be pursued.

Embryonic development from weeks 3 to 7 (5–9 weeks menstrual age), and the following 2 weeks of the fetal period, are the most sensitive times for the development of major malformations. It is during this time that development progresses from a trilaminar embryo through organogenesis. For any particular teratogenic agent, the effect is generally limited to a critical period during these weeks of pregnancy. Because formation of many structures occurs simultaneously, drugs which act during a short critical period may result in characteristic multiple malformations which may be described as a "syndrome." On the other hand, the teratogenic effect may be confined to a single structure or organ system and exert different effects over longer periods of time. An example of this is the teratogenic effect of androgens on the female fetus. These are confined to the genital tract but may vary with the gestational age and duration of exposure. The cellular mechanism by which many animal and most human teratogens cause structural malformations during embryogenesis has not been well defined. The limited number of drugs and chemicals which have been established as embryotoxic in humans are listed in Table 2.1.

Throughout the remainder of pregnancy (weeks 12 to term by menstrual age) there is continued growth and development of fetal organs, which may be affected by environmental exposure. It is during this time that drugs may cause generalized growth retardation. Most often this is due to a maternal pharmacologic effect which results in decreasing uterine blood flow. Toward the end of pregnancy, direct pharmacologic effects of drugs on the fetus may be noted by the mother (e.g., diminished fetal movement following administration of sedatives) or detected by biophysical monitoring (e.g., fetal heart rate changes in response to cardioactive drugs). In addition to the anticipated effects of drugs, fetal complications of drug therapy may also occur. For example, an increased frequency of stillbirth in patients taking warfarin derivatives is thought to be due to the anticoagulant effects on the fetus, resulting in hemorrhagic complications. Oxidant drugs have been reported to cause hemolysis and hydrops fetalis in male fetuses with severe G-6-PD deficiency.

Drugs administered very late in pregnancy or during labor may have pharmacologic properties which impair neonatal adaption or complicate neonatal care. Effects of central nervous system depressants administered shortly prior to delivery may be observed during the first hours or days of life. Drugs that compete with bilirubin binding may increase the risk of developing kernicterus during the early neonatal period when glucuronyl transferase is not well developed (sulfonamides and salicylates).

In the following section, groups of pharmacologic agents having known or suspected fetal effects discussed, which are most frequently used during pregnancy in the practice of emergency medicine, are considered.

Table 2-1. Embryotoxic drugs in human pregnancy.

Psychotropic Drugs Thalidomide—characteristic syndrome limb reduction multiple malformations Alcohol—characteristic syndrome growth and developmental delay short palpebral fissure craniofacial and limb malformations	**Hormones** Androgens—masculinization of female fetus Progestins—masculinization of female fetus Estrogens—hypospadias in male fetus Diethylstilbestrol—vaginal adenosis Mullerian malformation
Anticonvulsants Hydantonin—characteristic syndrome growth and developmental delay craniofacial and limb malformation hypoplastic distal phalanges Tridione—characteristic syndrome developmental delay craniofacial malformation "V" shaped eyebrows	**Folic Acid Antogionists** Aminopterin—small stature craniofacial malformation Amethopterin—small stature
Anticoagulants Warfarin—characteristic syndrome nasal hypoplasia chondrodysplasia punctata	**Other Drugs** Methyl mercury—minimata disease Inorganic Iodide—goiter, hypothyroidism I^{131}—thyroid ablation

PHARMACOLOGIC AGENTS IN CURRENT CLINICAL USE

Antibiotics

Antibiotics are often required during pregnancy, most commonly for treatment of urinary tract infection. Teratogenicity in animals has been established for many antimicrobial agents; however, these effects have not been observed in humans. Among the agents available, penicillin and its derivatives are generally considered safe for use. Ototoxicity has been observed in a proportion of infants exposed to streptomycin. Although streptomycin is rarely used during pregnancy, this observation has led to some concern regarding the potential oxotoxic effect of aminoglycosides for the fetus. In addition to a risk of hepatocellular necrosis in the mother when tetracycline is administered parenterally during late pregnancy, this antibiotic becomes incorporated into the fetal teeth and bones during calcification. This causes staining of the teeth following *in utero* exposure, and it has been suggested that there may be an effect on bone growth. The "gray syndrome" observed in newborns following chloramphenicol therapy provides a relative contraindication to the use of this drug during late pregnancy. Drugs which compete with bilirubin for albumin binding sites (e.g., sulfonamides) should not be selected for use in late pregnancy. Oxidant drugs, such as nitrofurantoins, should be avoided in potentially G-6-PD deficient pregnancies.

Analgesics

Analgesic drugs are generally considered safe during pregnancy, but a tendency for inappropriate use to treat minor discomforts of pregnancy should be avoided. Salicylates have been suggested to be associated with an increased incidence of abortion. An association of these compounds with prolonged gestation has been observed. The potential adverse effect on platelet function, with attendant risk for the mother and fetus, appears to be the primary reason to avoid salicylates as a mild analgesic during pregnancy. Potent analgesics may have central nervous system depressant effects in the newborn when used during late pregnancy or shortly prior to delivery. Thus indication for the use of many of these agents should be carefully considered when labor is imminent. Reversibility of effects by narcotic antagonists is possible.

Anticoagulants

Warfarin derivatives, commonly used for chronic anticoagulation, have been associated with a specific pattern of embryotoxicity. This syndrome, which includes hypoplasia of the nasal bridge, chondrodysplasia punctata, and possible developmental delay, has been observed in infants exposed during the first trimester. The proportion of exposed infants who will be affected is not known but has been estimated to be as high as 50 percent.[10] The definition of a warfarin embryopathy syndrome, along with an increased risk of hemorrhagic complications when used during the third trimester, has resulted in this drug being considered contraindicated during pregnancy. Heparin, on the other hand, does not cross the placenta and has not been associated with adverse fetal effects. Thus, in spite of difficulty with administration of heparin on a chronic basis, it has become the anticoagulant of choice throughout pregnancy.

Anticonvulsants

A 2 to 3 fold increase in the frequency of malformations among children born to mothers with epilepsy, most especially facial clefts, has led to a suspicion of teratogenic effects of the commonly used anticonvulsants. The effect of the maternal disease or the genetic liability of the offspring of an epileptic has been difficult to separate from an effect of the drugs. The frequent use of multiple drugs to treat most patients with this disease has further compounded this problem.

Recently, specific malformation syndromes have been described in infants exposed to hydantoins and also to trimethadione. The prominent features of the fetal hydantoin syndrome include: mild to moderate growth deficiency of prenatal onset, mild developmental delay, a characteristic facial appearance (metopic ridging, ocular hypertelorism, broad nasal bridge, low set ears), and hypoplasia of the distal phalanges and nails[11] The proportion of affected infants has not been determined. One or more features of this syndrome may be seen in a large proportion of exposed pregnancies (possibly 30 percent or more), although the frequency of serious growth or developmental impairment is probably considerably lower. Manifestations of the tridione syndrome include mental deficiency, prenatal growth deficiency, characteristic facies ("V-shaped" eyebrows, mid-facial hypoplasia, abnormal ears) and a variety of associated malformations.[12] The proportion of exposed pregnancies which will be affected has not been defined. An increased frequency of spontaneous abortions among women who use this drug has also been suggested. These findings have led to the recommendation that women in the reproductive years who are taking hydantoin or tridione should consider a trial of discontinuing therapy or changing to other drugs prior to becoming pregnant.

Hormones

Continuation of chronic adrenal corticosteroid therapy for certain maternal diseases is frequently necessary during pregnancy and, on occasion, acute steroid therapy may be indicated. Early reports suggesting an increased frequency of cleft palate in exposed human pregnancies were supported by data establishing a relationship between these agents and facial clefts in certain strains of animals. Thus, there has been a reluctance to use corticosteroids during early human pregnancy. The actual level of risk of clefts, if increased, appears to be quite low. Because palatine closure occurs by the eighth week in humans (10 weeks after the last menstrual period) there does not seem to be substantial concern regarding teratogenesis beyond this point. Transient neonatal adrenal insufficiency after chronic *in utero* exposure is a very unusual occurrence, although at risk neonates should be closely observed for this complication. Because of the serious nature of many of the maternal diseases which require chronic steroid therapy or the emergent situations requiring acute short term therapy, the risk/benefit considerations usually favor maternal treatment.

Non-steroidal estrogens, specifically diethylstilbestrol, have been shown to cause Mullerian malformations (cervical hood, adenosis of the vagina) in exposed females. This association was first made when a number of young women with this history were found to have clear cell carcinoma of the vagina and/or cervix.[13] With aggressive ascertainment and careful follow-up, the finding of adenosis in exposed women has been determined to be quite frequent, although the risk of development of genital malignancy appears to be very low. When diethylstilbestrol is used as a postcoital contraceptive, it is mandatory that the diagnosis of pregnancy be excluded. Administration of this drug shortly prior to conception has not been shown to cause adverse effects in subsequent conceptions. Nevertheless, some physicians restrict this therapy to those patients who feel they would terminate a pregnancy if the postcoital contraceptive effect failed.

The male and female external genitalia differentiate from the same primitive embryologic structure; i.e., genital tubercle, urogenital folds, and labioscrotal swellings. Differentiation of the male external genitalia occurs during weeks 8 through 13. This is under the influence of testosterone produced by the fetal testis. Maternally administered testosterone or other androgenic steroids (including certain progestogens) during this critical period will cause masculinization of the external genitalia of a female fetus. Depending upon the dose and duration of exposure, effects may range from varying degrees of fusion of the labioscrotal folds to clitoromegaly. The latter abnormality may occur from exposure even after the 13th week. In addition to the potential for masculinization of the female genitalia by progestational drugs, a number of these agents, as well as estrogens, have been associated with the development of hypospadias in males. Retrospective and prospective studies have shown conflicting results regarding an association of congenital heart defects, limb reduction deformities, and the VACTERL association of anomalies (Vertebral, Anal, Cardiac, Tracheoesophageal fistula, Renal, and Limb) with the use of progestational agents during early pregnancy. On the basis of this suspicion, it seems prudent to discontinue the previously common practice of administering progestational drugs to induce withdrawal bleeding as a form of very early pregnancy testing.

Psychotropic Drugs

Several case reports of cardiac defects (Epstein anomaly) in infants exposed to lithium have raised a suspicion of teratogenicity of this drug. Subsequent surveillance of babies born after lithium exposure has confirmed a higher than expected frequency of cardiac malformations. It is likely that this agent is teratogenic; however, the risk of malformations has not been defined. Several large retrospective studies have shown conflicting results in regard to possible teratogenicity due to minor tranquilizers, specifically meprobamate and chlordiazepoxide. Two case control studies suggest a several fold increased risk of cleft lip and cleft palate following intrauterine exposure to diazepam. In spite of the suspicion of this association, a causal relationship has not been established with confidence. An association of congenital heart defects and amphetamine exposure has also been suggested. Notably congenital heart defects and oral facial clefts are among the most common major defects observed as isolated malformations. Further prospective studies are required before a causal inference can be drawn regarding a low level of teratogenicity between the particular psychotropic drugs and these defects. Nevertheless, because these suspicions have been raised, but also because these drugs are generally not absolutely necessary for maternal health, prescribing them for women in the first trimester should be avoided.

Antihistamines and Antinauseants

In addition to viral upper respiratory infections, the normal congestion of the mucous membranes during pregnancy frequently results in symptoms for which patients request antihistamine therapy. This group of drugs has had widespread use during pregnancy without demonstrable adverse fetal effects. They are, in fact, commonly employed as a mild sedative for patients who have difficulty sleeping due to minor discomforts of pregnancy.

Recently there has been a great deal of adverse publicity regarding a possible association of birth defects with the antinauseant (Bendectin) most commonly used during pregnancy. Considering the widespread use of this drug during pregnancy and the frquency of major malformations, it is not surprising that instances of malformation would occur following this treatment. Previously, a number of retrospective and prospective studies had not demonstrated an association of antinauseants with birth defects or poor pregnancy outcome.[14,15] The continued reinforcement of a possible teratogenic effect of these drugs in the lay press has caused a great deal of parental anxiety and reluctance on the part of physicians to treat this pregnancy related symptom. Changes in eating patterns and dietary constituents may alleviate symptoms in many cases when they are mild. Nevertheless, the available scientific evidence supports the safety of this therapy when symptoms are persistent and interfere with normal nutrition. Certainly, the occasional patient with such complications as dehydration, electrolytic imbalance, weight loss, and esophageal tears requires hospitalization, and nutritional as well as pharmacologic management.

CONCLUSION

In very few clinical situations can the physician either assure a couple of the safety of a drug for their pregnancy or give them accurate scientific information regarding a known risk of teratogenicity. Increasing concern regarding the effects not only of drugs but of other environmental exposures has led some to withhold therapy from pregnant women in almost all circumstances. It seems, however, that between this position and one in which patients or physicians use drugs to alleviate minor symptoms of pregnancy, a more moderate approach should prevail. Knowledge of the general principles discussed in this article as well as the available scientific information should be considered when establishing a risk/benefit ratio for treating the pregnant woman. Quite clearly the known or possible adverse effects for the mother and/or fetus arising from failure to treat may outweigh the uncertainty about the safety of a drug in the truly emergency situation.

REFERENCES

1. Doering PL, Stewart RB: The extent and character of drug consumption during pregnancy, JAMA 239:843, 1978.
2. Heinonen OP, Sloane D, Shapiro S: Major malformations. p. 65. Kaufman DW, Ed: In Birth Defects and Drugs in Pregnancy. Publishing Sciences Group, Littleton MA, 1977.
3. Wilson JG: Embryotoxicity of drugs in man. p. 309. In Wilson JG, Fraser FC: Handbook of Teratology. Vol. 1. New York, Plenum Press, 1977.
4. Van Thiel DH, Ross GT, Lipsett MB: Trophoblastic neoplasms. Science 169:1326, 1970.

5. Oakley GP, Flynt JW: Increased prevalence of Down's syndrome (mongolism) among the offspring of women treated with ovulation-inducing agents. Teratology 5:264, 1972.
6. Harlap S, Shiono PH: Alcohol, smoking, and incidence of spontaneous abortions in the first and second trimester. Lancet 173, 1980.
7. Kline J, Shrout P, Stein Z, et al: Drinking during pregnancy and spontaneous abortion. Lancet 176, 1980.
8. Mennuti MT: Drugs and chemical risks to the fetus: occupational hazards for medical personnel. p. 41. In Schwarz RH and Yaffe SJ Eds: Drug and Chemical Risks to the Fetus and Newborn. Alan R. Liss, Inc., New York, 1980.
9. Ericson A, Kallen B: Survey of infants born in 1973 or 1975 to Swedish women working in operating rooms during their pregnancies. Anesth Anal 58:302, 1979.
10. Hall JG, Shaul WL: Multiple congenital anomalies associated with oral anticoagulants. Am J Obstet Gynecol 127:191, 1977.
11. Hanson JW, Smith DW: The fetal hydantoin syndrome. J Pediat 87:285, 1975.
12. Remigo PA, Grinvalsky HT: Osteogenesis imperfecta congenita. Am J Dis Child 119:524, 1970.
13. Herbst AL, Scully RE: Adenocarcinoma of the vagina in adolescence: a report of 7 cases including 6 clear cell carcinoma. Cancer 25:745, 1970.
14. Milkovich L, Van Den Berg BJ: An evaluation of the teratogenicity of certain antinauseant drugs. Am J Obstet Gynecol 125:244, 1975.
15. Heinonen OP, Sloane D, Shapirto S: Antinauseants, antihistamines, and phenothiazines. p. 322. In Kaufman DW, Ed: Birth Defects and Drugs in Pregnancy. Publishing Sciences Group, Littleton MA 1977.

SUGGESTED READINGS

Bergsma D, Ed: Birth Defects Compendium. 2nd Ed. The National Foundation—March of Dimes. Alan R. Liss, Inc., New York, 1979.

Berkowitz RL and Coustan DR: The Handbook for Drugs in Pregnancy. Little, Brown (In press).

Kaufman DW, Ed: Birth Defects and Drugs in Pregnancy. Publishing Sciences Group, Littleton MA, 1977.

Shepard TH: Catalog of Teratogenic Agents. The Johns Hopkins University Press, Baltimore, 1973.

Smith DW: Recognizable Patterns of Human Malformation. 2nd Ed. W.B. Saunders, Philadelphia, 1976.

Warkany J: Congenital Malformations. Year Book Medical Publishers, Chicago, 1971.

3 The Acute Abdomen in Pregnancy

James R. Huey, Jr.

Acute abdominal disease during pregnancy is rare, but when a patient with these two conditions presents to an emergency room, she should be handled as expeditiously as possible. Most acute nonobstetric abdominal crises occur no more frequently in the gravid woman than in the nongravid, with a few exceptions such as urinary tract disease. In a pregnant patient, acute abdominal pain is a source of special concern because two lives are involved; both will be affected by the course of management. Isotope studies, radiographs, or surgical procedures should not be taken lightly because of the added risk to the fetus or the risk of causing premature labor. Therefore, one needs to be as certain as possible of the diagnosis prior to proceeding with treatment. The evaluation of the acute abdomen during pregnancy is more difficult because of the enlarging uterus and other physiologic changes. Certain problems of the very young or old female can be excluded; by definition, we are dealing with women in the reproductive years.

The emergency or family practice physician should work closely with the surgeon and/or obstetrician whenever possible in evaluating the pregnant patient presenting with an acute abdomen. In this chapter, the diagnosis and management of more common conditions presenting in the gravida as an acute abdomen are stressed.

Prior to the discussion of specific conditions, diagnosis of pregnancy, physiologic changes during pregnancy, and the approach to evaluation of abdominal pain in pregnancy are covered. Physicians with a true interest in delivering emergency care have been instrumental in finding ways to a more rapid evaluation time, which is often critical, leading to better diagnosis and proper treatment of the gravida with benefits both to the patient and to her fetus.

DIAGNOSIS OF PREGNANCY

The physician working in the emergency room is frequently at a disadvantage with no records at fingertip, as the patient presents in a state of anxiety secondary to pain, giving only the history she feels is pertinent to the pain. She may overlook or even be unaware that she is pregnant. It is especially important for the emergency room physician to consider the possibility of pregnancy when examining and treating females in the reproductive years. Diagnostic procedures and treatment, or lack of treatment, may have far-reaching effects for the developing fetus (Chapter 2).

Table 3.1 lists several signs and symptoms useful as clues to suspect pregnancy when evaluating an emergency patient (see also Chapter 1). Most often, the patient will give the history of being pregnant or attempting conception if she is questioned. The time of the last menstrual flow, if the woman is previously regular and not using hormonal birth control, will give a good indication. If a woman who was previously having spontaneous, cyclic menstruation misses the second period, the likelihood is high that she is pregnant.

In some patients, the history will not be obtained as easily because of anxiety or hostility directed at the physician. This may be especially true of the adolescent patient not fully understanding the importance of a complete history. Women often find physicians condescending, judgmental, and unsympathetic in their lack of comprehension of women's problems, and rightly fear not being understood by their physician. "The gynecologic history requires that the woman reveal her actions and feelings, past and present, as they relate to sex. Because of the wide variation in ethical and religious teachings together with a legal code reflecting the sexual mores of an earlier era, a woman faces an unknown doctor with apprehension about how she will be received. If she has had an unpleasant experience in the past, she may be reluctant to be honest with the doctor." [1]

Two points must be kept in mind by the physician seeing emergency patients. Uterine bleeding felt to be menstruation is not infrequently seen following conception. The flow is usually light and of shorter duration than what is considered a normal menses. Speert and Guttmacher [2] reported vaginal bleeding in 8 percent of pregnancies on or before the fortieth day after conception. Overall, bleeding during pregnancy was reported three times as frequent among multiparas as among primigravidas.

The second point is that conception may occur prior to menstruation. This is notoriously true of nursing mothers, but may also occur in very young,

Table 3-1. Pregnancy signs and symptoms.

Amenorrhea	Fetal movement
Breast tenderness	Fetal heart tones
Nausea	Uterine enlargement
Urinary frequency	Cervical color
Fatigue	Cervical consistency
Uterine softness	Discoloration of vaginal mucosa

sexually active girls. This is especially a problem as unplanned pregnancies are occurring at a continuously rising rate in younger and younger teenagers. Pregnant adolescents, and especially those who are poor, nonwhite, or both, represent high-risk individuals and are more likely to be seen in an emergency room.

Urinary frequency is a common symptom of early pregnancy because of pressure of the enlarging uterus on the bladder. This symptom is often attributed to the problem causing the acute abdomen and usually does not ring a bell in the emergency room. Urinary frequency and nocturia with a normal urinalysis should raise suspicion of pelvic mass.

Easy fatigability is a frequent complaint of early pregnancy. Often multigravidas will suspect they have conceived by this early symptom. Again, as a vague symptom, this is attributed to the origin of the acute abdomen.

Nausea of pregnancy is an often talked-about symptom of the first trimester; but in reality, it is probably less frequent in occurrence than is urinary frequency and the complaint of excessive fatigue.

Changes seen and felt on pelvic examination may lead to a suspicion of pregnancy. The vaginal mucosa frequently appears dark-bluish or purple or congested (Chadwick's sign). During the first 2 months of pregnancy, the cervix becomes progressively more soft and cyanotic. Softening of the isthmus, between the cervix and the body of the uterus, may be very marked after the first month (Hegar's sign). After the first 6 weeks of pregnancy, the fundus begins to enlarge and soften; this enlargement can be appreciated by pelvic examination, leading to the suspicion of pregnancy.

Late findings to confirm pregnancy would include fetal movement at 16 to 20 weeks and fetal heart tones heard as early as 12 to 14 weeks from conception with the hand-held ultrasound and with the fetoscope by 18 to 20 weeks. With the presence of real-time ultrasound as a back-up procedure in some emergency rooms, pregnancy can be detected as early as 6 weeks with careful scanning.

Even with the presence of all the support possible, the bottom line is that unless the physician has a high index of suspicion of pregnancy when evaluating a woman in the reproductive years, the diagnosis will not be made.

PHYSIOLOGIC CHANGES DURING PREGNANCY

Normal, expected, physiologic changes which occur with each pregnancy need to be understood when evaluating the gravida with an acute abdomen. Most organ systems have some change in function during pregnancy. Only a minority of these changes are related to the enlarging uterus. Most changes are brought about under the effects of placental or ovarian hormones from the pregnancy. The reader with a desire for an indepth review of these changes is referred to *Physiologic Changes During Pregnancy: The Mother,* by Chester Martin, M.D.[3]

Reproductive Tract Anatomical Changes

The uterus increases from approximately 60 g before pregnancy to 1200 g at term. The volume at term is nearly 5 liters in a normal, singleton pregnancy and greater with hydramnios or multiple pregnancy. The cervix and lower genital tract become hyperemic, which accounts for softening and cyanosis of the cervix and vagina. These changes are responsible for transudation of fluid into the vaginal lumen.

Functional Changes of the Reproductive Tract

Uterine contractions occurring at a rate of 3 to 4 per minute at ovulation are effectively suppressed to a great degree during pregnancy, at least in part by progesterone. During the first 30 weeks of gestation, the uterine contractions are small, generally confined to only a local area of uterine muscle. Some will reach higher intensity, spreading over much of the uterus, and are called Braxton-Hicks contractions. These contractions increase gradually in frequency after the first 30 weeks, reaching a rate of 1 per hour. They increase, in both intensity and frequency, the last 10 weeks of gestation. As term nears, the interspaced small and large contractions evolve into strong, well-coordinated, rhythmic contractions as the transition from pre-labor to labor is made.[4] Along with this change in uterine activity, there is an increase in the sensitivity of the myometrium to oxytocic agents.

Uterine blood flow progressively increases from approximately 75 ml per minute at 16 weeks to over 500 ml per minute at term. Blood flow to the uterus increases as rapidly as its growth during pregnancy. By ultrasonic studies, the average volume of the placenta increases from 60 ml at 10 weeks to 950 ml at term.[5]

Cardiovascular Changes

The apex of the heart is moved upward, slightly left, and rotated forward, displacing the heart into a more transverse position by diaphragm elevation during pregnancy. Cardiac volume is increased. Systolic murmurs are frequently present, caused by increased flow rates. Premature beats are more frequent with pregnancy.

Cardiac output increases by about 40 percent from nonpregnant values, peaking probably near the middle of pregnancy. During late pregnancy, cardiac output in the supine position is lower than in the lateral position. The increase is due to both an increase in heart rate and increase in stroke volume. Arterial blood pressure falls slightly during pregnancy, with a decrease in total peripheral vascular resistance. Plasma volume expands by 50 percent, peaking at 34 weeks.

The total volume of red cells increases, but because of a relatively greater increase in plasma volume causing a dilutional effect, there is a fall in hemoglobin concentration and the hematocrit. At 30 to 32 weeks, the lowest values are seen in the hemoglobin and hematocrit, with slight rise in healthy gravidas as term approaches. An increase in polymorphonuclear leucocytes raises the total white blood cell count to about 10,500 per cubic millimeter.

The platelet count is reduced by hemodilution, while fibrinogen increases as term is approached, up to 50 percent above the pre-pregnant state. Fibrin degradation product levels rise in normal pregnancy.

Respiratory Changes in Pregnancy

The diaphragm rises nearly 4 cm with a flare of the lower ribs which reduces the residual volume. The respiratory center is more sensitive, increasing in some a desire to breathe and giving a feeling of breathlessness, especially with any activity. These findings have been mistaken for pathologic dyspnea.

Urinary Changes in Pregnancy

Because of hyperemia and hypertrophy, the kidneys may be slightly enlarged during pregnancy. The ureter course is tortuous, because of dilatation and elongation. Both of these changes produce a slowing of urine flow, which contributes to the predisposition to urinary tract infections during pregnancy.

The bladder is progressively elevated by the uterus, and the trigone undergoes hyperplasia and hypertrophy. The stretching of the trigone may produce incompetence of the ureterovesical valves, also predisposing to urinary tract infections.

Renal blood flow and glomerular filtration rates are elevated at about 50 percent above nonpregnant values. This in turn leads to elevated renal clearance of many substances, with a resultant fall in serum urea and creatinine levels to two-thirds of their pre-pregnant values. Results of function studies must be evaluated in light of normal pregnancy values.

Gastrointestinal Changes in Pregnancy

As the uterus increases in size, the lower esophageal sphincter may be displaced into the thorax along with upward stomach displacement, leading to gastroesophageal reflux. Both gastric tone and motility are reduced, with resultant longer retention of food, thus increasing the danger of regurgitation and aspiration, especially under general anesthesia. Motility is reduced throughout the intestinal tract. Constipation is a common complaint. The gallbladder, likewise, is hypotonic and empties poorly. Gallstone formation is favored during pregnancy because of increased bile concentration and incomplete emptying of the gallbladder.

Musculoskeletal Changes in Pregnancy

Low back pain, and rarely lumbar or sacral nerve root irritation, may occur in late pregnancy because of an increased lumbar lordosis and weakened joint ligamentous support.

GENERAL EVALUATION OF ABDOMINAL PAIN

The amount of stimuli required to evoke pain varies greatly among people; the pregnant state is no exception. Detailed information concerning the onset, location, quality, duration, aggravating and relieving conditions, and associated symptoms is necessary for an accurate evaluation of the acute abdomen in pregnancy. However, in pregnancy, the evaluation of the acute abdomen is more difficult because of added problems specifically related to pregnancy. The classic clinical signs are changed or masked by the enlarging uterus, altering anatomical and topographical landmarks, concealing muscular responses by stretching the abdominal wall, and making palpation of intraabdominal masses more difficult.[6]

Abdominal pain of a regular periodic nature is generally from the uterus, but may also be of ureteral, intestinal, or tubal origin. If the uterus is large enough to be palpated and contracts with each episode of pain, the origin is found. If the uterus is not contracting, or the maximum intensity of pain is not with uterine contractions, a search for other sources of pain should be carried out.

SPECIFIC CONDITIONS CAUSING THE ACUTE ABDOMEN

If pain is not related to the uterus and is from a nonobstetric source, but coincident with pregnancy, other diagnoses must be entertained. Table 3.2 lists conditions giving rise to acute abdominal symptoms that may present during

Table 3-2. Concurrent diagnoses of pregnancy.

1. Persistent vomiting
2. Inflammatory or ulcerative gastrointestinal disease
3. Ectopic pregnancy
4. Threatened abortion
5. Septic abortion
6. Renal stones
7. Cholecystitis
8. Pancreatitis
9. Pyelitis
10. Fibroid degeneration
11. Uterine rupture
12. Appendicitis
13. Meckel's diverticulitis
14. Torsion of ovary, ovarian cyst, or fibroids
15. Pelvic peritonitis
16. Acute pelvic inflammatory disease
17. Intestinal obstruction
18. Traumatic injuries in pregnancy

pregnancy or the puerperium. Several of these conditions will be covered in this chapter; others are covered elsewhere in this book.

The incidence of acute abdomen during pregnancy is difficult to define. The reported frequency varies, depending upon the type of population the hospital serves, geographical location of the hospital, and its referral base. Hospitals with active emergency room services have larger numbers of trauma and pregnancy cases. Hospitals with large, indigent populations appear to report more inflammatory disease. Garry (1957) reported 32 laparotomies among 17,000 pregnancies. In his review, 27 carried full term, 3 required hysterectomies, and 2 delivered prematurely.[7] In 1965, Shnider and Webster reported that of 9,073 pregnancies, 147 required some type of surgery.[8]

Appendicitis

Shnider reported on a cooperative study of 60,912 pregnancies which included 50 appendectomies.[8] Cavanagh states that appendicitis complicates 1 pregnancy in approximately 1,200, the same incidence as in the nonpregnant population.[9] Many surveys of appendicitis complicating pregnancy have appeared in the literature, with the frequency nearly always around 1 case per 1,000 deliveries. The reported incidence of finding normal appendices following laparotomy for suspected appendicitis varies from 25 to 50 percent, with these numbers felt justified by all authors.

As previously mentioned, as the uterus enlarges, the cecum and appendix are displaced upward, laterally, and sometimes posteriorly, altering the clinical picture.[10] The normal leukocytosis of pregnancy, and the not uncommon right round ligament pain as stretching occurs, may further confuse the picture.

Delaying surgery will lead to higher incidence of morbidity and mortality, as the inflammatory process in pregnancy may be more severe and lead to more rapid perforation. The more intense the disease, and thus the inflammatory reaction, the more likely to be associated with premature labor from uterine irritation. Hoffman and Suzuki [11] reported an increase in the premature labor rate from 11 percent to 35 percent with the advancement of the disease from only appendicitis to generalized peritonitis.

Diagnosis. The pain usually begins periumbilically and progresses to the right lower quadrant, especially in the first trimester. As pregnancy advances, this progress may be higher on the right side, reaching under the costal margin by 38 weeks.[12] Nausea and vomiting are common pregnancy symptoms, but if not present before the onset of pain, should be considered significant. The tenderness may be very mild, especially with a posterior appendix, until late in the course. As pregnancy advances, the pain should be expected to be higher on the right side, and may be at McBurney's point only during the first 2 to 3 months of pregnancy. Even though the white count is elevated in pregnancy, further rise and especially a left shift should be considered significant.

Kark states that it is always prudent to suspect acute appendicitis in a pregnant woman with right sided pain; if after a few hours observation, the clinical picture is still suggestive, exploratory laparotomy should be undertaken without delay.[6] Present in 1.5 percent of the population,[13] Meckel's diverticulum may present with the same symptoms.

Urinary Tract Infection

The frequency of urinary tract infections and their relationship to poor outcome in pregnancy make this an important part of the evaluation of any pregnant patient with an acute abdomen. All women with asymptomatic bacteriuria in pregnancy should be treated.[14] This refers to positive cultures in gravidas who have no urinary tract symptoms. Numerous studies have reported on the incidence of urinary tract infection in asymptomatic women, with an average rate of 5 to 6 percent in both pregnant and nonpregnant sexually active patients of the same age group.[14]

Kass reported that 40 percent of his gravidas who had untreated asymptomatic bacteriuria developed symptomatic urinary tract infections later in pregnancy.[15] Harris has reported that effective antimicrobial treatment of bacteriuria early in pregnancy will substantially lower the subsequent incidence of overt, symptomatic urinary tract infection and its potentially disastrous complications.[16] Pyelonephritis occurs in 1 to 2 percent of all gravidas and is seen more commonly in primigravidas. There frequently will have been a history of lower tract infection or asymptomatic bacteriuria earlier in the pregnancy.[1] Presenting complaints include urgency, frequency, dysuria, flank pain, chills, anorexia, vomiting, and high fever. The differential diagnosis must include ureteral calculus, lobar pneumonia, acute appendicitis, and cholecystitis. The treatment must be started immediately and aggressively to lower the associated increased incidence of spontaneous abortion, premature labor, and stillbirth.

Pyelonephritis during pregnancy requires hospitalization and hydration along with antibiotic treatment. The treatment will not be effective without adequate drainage of the renal pelvis and ureter. This seldom requires ureteral catheterization and is usually treated by Trendelenburg position with the affected side up.

Diagnosis. Symptomatic patients present as non-pregnant patients present, with the exception that frequency cannot be relied upon as a pathologic symptom in pregnancy. Lindheimer and Katz feel strongly that bladder catheterization has little place in modern obstetrics, and prefer suprapubic aspiration for diagnostic purposes.[14]

Treatment should include, for the initial episode, 2 weeks of active antibiotic therapy, followed by repeat urine colony count and cultures in all patients monthly throughout pregnancy. Tetracycline and chloramphenicol are contraindicated in pregnancy. The sulfonamides should not be used during the last 4 to 6 weeks of pregnancy because of the interference in the neonate with bilirubin transport. Patients with a repeated resistant organism, either symptomatic or asymptomatic, should be suppressed with some antibiotic for the remainder of the pregnancy.

Renal or Ureteral Stones

Urinary tract stones are frequently silent during pregnancy because of the dilated system. The occurrence is reported at 0.1 to 0.3 percent in pregnancy.[17] Harris and Dunnihoo reported ureteral stones occurring twice as frequently as renal stones. Most of the stones found in pregnancy are of infectious origin and contain calcium. Folger reported that renal calculi were the most common cause requiring hospitalization of abdominal pain in pregnancy.[18] Coe reviewed 78 women with a diagnosis of nephrolithiasis and pregnancy occurring during or following the condition.[19] He found no prejudicial effect on pregnancy except for increased incidence of urinary tract infections. Also, pregnancy exerted no visible effect on stone disease.

Diagnosis. When not silent during pregnancy, many of the stones are found in relation to urinary tract infection. Symptoms include severe costovertebral angle colicky pain, often radiating down the ureter path and to the groin. This is usually associated with urgency, frequency, and hematuria.

Ovarian Cysts

Ovarian tumors of any type are prone to hemorrhage, torsion, suppuration, tumor previa with dystocia, or rupture during pregnancy. They may demand immediate surgery. If, unilaterally, a free, mobile, round, cystic, smooth, less than 6 cm cyst is found, it is likely to be the physiologic corpus luteum of pregnancy. Management will consist of repeat exams every 2 to 3 weeks to insure no further increase in size. At the Mayo Clinic, the incidence of operative ovarian disease in pregnancy was 1 case in every 536 deliveries.[20] Booth reported 1 ovarian tumor diagnosed for every 591 deliveries.[21] The incidence of ovarian neoplasms complicating pregnancy is 0.1 percent; the frequency of an accident in the immediate postpartum period is as high as 40 percent. Benign cystic teratomas account for between 12 and 50 percent of these in various series.[20,21] One-third of these are serous or pseudomucinous cystadenomas with significant malignant potential. The frequency of seeing solid ovarian tumors during pregnancy is 0.01 percent, with two-thirds being malignant.[1]

Diagnosis. Ovarian tumors usually remain asymptomatic until they undergo an accident such as torsion and cause an acute abdomen requiring surgery. Cavanagh reports a torsion incidence of ovarian tumors in pregnancy of 12 percent. The clinical picture includes intermittent colicky pain, usually unilateral in the lower abdomen. A cyst trapped in the pelvis may cause severe backache. Late signs include peritonitis and fever. (These signs of rupture demand immediate surgery.) The abdomen becomes rigid with muscle guarding, tenderness, and rebound. Change in the blood count is a late finding. Ultrasound may outline the mass as well as detail its internal character.

Degenerating Fibroid

Uterine myomas (fibroids) may be submucous (beneath the endometrium), subserous (beneath the uterine serosa), or intramural (located in the myometrium). The subserous or submucous fibroid may be pedunculated. As pregnancy advances, the myomas increase in size under the influence of estrogen, sometimes markedly. They may undergo torsion, if pedunculated, followed by necrosis. Submucous myomas may become infected postpartum or after an abortion. As the myomas grow with pregnancy, they may outdistance the blood supply and undergo hemorrhagic infarction or "red degeneration." Pelvic or cervical myomas may also obstruct labor.[22]

Diagnosis. A degenerating myoma causes focal pain, overlying abdominal tenderness to palpation and occasionally a low grade fever and leukocytosis. When severe, especially with infarction, the differential diagnosis may include torsion of the adnexa, appendicitis, ureteral stone, abruption, or pyelonephritis. Myomectomy during pregnancy should be avoided if possible, and then limited to the pedunculated variety. Myomas usually regress rapidly following delivery. Ultrasound examination may be of some value in the diagnosis, depending upon the location in relation to the uterine contents.

Cholecystitis

As with the nonpregnant population, pregnant patients with gallbladder disease usually are obese and have a previous history that is suggestive of gallbladder disease. Predisposing factors for aggravation of the disease during pregnancy include hypotonia of the ductal system, decreased emptying time, hypercholesterolemia, and changes in bile excretion. The reported incidence in pregnancy is 0.02 percent, with 90 percent or more having associated cholelithiasis.[1] If at all possible, surgery should be avoided until after pregnancy because of the complication rate. The patients should be treated with a bland diet, low in fat, and antispasmodics.

Diagnosis. The symptoms of gall bladder disease are typical symptoms of the nonpregnant patient, including epigastric distress and attacks of biliary colic. The right upper quadrant colicky pain radiates to the subscapular area. Acute attacks are accompanied by leukocytosis, fever, tachycardia, and a tender right upper quadrant mass. Jaundice also may be seen in pregnancy.

Pancreatitis

Pancreatitis in pregnancy has a reported incidence of from 1 in 3,800 pregnancies to 1 in 11,467, and is considered to be extremely hazardous for the mother and fetus.[23] The same clinical picture is presented as in the nonpregnant state. The acute attacks are survived and management is conservative. Recurrent attacks during pregnancy are common.[24] There is no indication for therapeutic abortion; conversely, any surgical intervention, including induction of labor, should be delayed as long as possible while medical treatment is underway.[23]

Diagnosis. A high index of suspicion is required, as the presence of an enlarged uterus may make it impossible to localize findings to the pancreas. The serum amylase rises and falls rapidly and may be normal by 72 hours, whereas the serum lipase rises slower and remains elevated longer. The elevation is higher than in other conditions causing an acute abdomen. Symptoms include severe upper abdominal pain, vomiting, fever, distention, and often severe boring pain radiating through the midback. In the first trimester, hyperemesis is included in the differential, while later it may appear as a perforated ulcer. Severe cases progress to shock.[24]

The aim of treatment is to avoid surgery if possible and to give the pancreas nearly complete rest. Treatment includes a broad spectrum antibiotic, nasogastric suction, and an anticholinergic agent. Demerol is helpful for relief of the severe pain.

TRAUMA DURING PREGNANCY

The subject of trauma during pregnancy is large, with many excellent literature reviews on such specific conditions as gunshot wounds or automobile accident injuries. An excellent book on the subject, published in 1979, entitled *Trauma in Pregnancy* and edited by H. J. Buchsbaum,[25] should be available to those who work emergency rooms where trauma is seen. As reviewed previously, the physiologic responses and anatomy are changed with pregnancy, giving rise to altered signs, symptoms, and laboratory values for both disease and injury. "The physician called upon to attend a pregnant trauma victim must remember that he does in fact have two patients, and a thorough understanding of the anatomic and physiologic alterations caused by pregnancy is essential if the best interests of both mother and fetus are to be served." [26]

In a study by Peckman and King,[27] the three major causes of accidental injury in a pregnant population were vehicular accidents, falls, and piercing instruments. They found no greater freuqncy in any trimester. In the first trimester, trauma seems to have no adverse effect on the pregnancy.[28]

In general, hemorrhagic shock and anoxia must be reversed as rapidly as possible in the mother to prevent any adverse effect upon the fetus. During trauma, the mother will maintain her own homeostasis at the expense of the uterus and fetus, with a disproportionately more severe fetal effect.

The most common penetrating injury is a gunshot wound. As would be expected with a growing uterus, the incidence of uterine injury is low in the first trimester and increases with advancing gestation. White reported a threefold decreased maternal mortality associated with gunshot wounds in the gravida as compared to the nonpregnant patient.[6] With all abdominal gunshot wounds, Buchsbaum recommends early exploration in pregnant patients. The changes of the abdominal response to injury caused by pregnancy may lead to misdiagnosis or delay, with irreversible damage occurring.

The pregnant trauma patient must be cared for as any victim, but possibly at a more rapid rate when the fetus is in jeopardy. Cruikshank [26] lists several complicating factors that the physician must keep in mind when caring for a pregnant trauma victim.

1. The fact that the patient is pregnant may alter the pattern of severity of the injury.

2. The pregnancy may alter the signs and symptoms of the injury and the results of laboratory tests used in diagnosis.

3. The management of the trauma victim needs to be modified to accommodate and preserve the physiologic changes induced by pregnancy.

4. The injury may have initiated or have been complicated by pathologic conditions peculiar to pregnancy (e.g., abruptio placenta, amniotic fluid embolism, ruptured uterus), or a pregnancy-related disease may occur coincidental to trauma and thus complicate the diagnosis and therapy (e.g., eclampsia complicating possible head trauma).

SUMMARY

In this chapter, the diagnosis and management of some nonobstetrical causes of acute abdominal disease complicating pregnancy have been reviewed. The physician must keep in mind that when dealing with a woman in the reproductive years, she may be pregnant; and if pregnant, certain physiologic alterations are occurring which may alter her response to disease and alter the expected response to treatment. When treating a pregnant patient, we have two lives which may be affected. Diagnostic procedures benign for the mother may prove detrimental to the fetus.

REFERENCES

1. Gray MJ, Van Buren HC: The reproductive years. p. 144. In Romney SL, Ed: Gynecology and Obstetrics: The Health Care of Women. McGraw-Hill, New York, 1975.
2. Speert H, Guttmacher AF: Frequency and significance of bleeding in early pregnancy. JAMA 155:712, 1954.
3. Martin C: Physiologic changes during pregnancy. p. 141. In Quilligan EJ, Kretchmer N, Eds: Fetal and Maternal Medicine. John Wiley and Sons, New York, 1980.
4. Caldeyro-Barcia R, Alvarez H, Poseiro J: Normal and abnormal uterine contractility in labor. Triangle 2:41, 1955.
5. Hellman LM, Kobayashi M, Tolles WE, Cromb E: Ultrasonic studies on the volumetric growth of the human placenta. Am J Obstet Gynecol 108:740, 1970.
6. Kark AE: Acute abdominal emergencies. p. 238–248. In Rovinsky JJ, Guttmacher AF, Eds: Medical, Surgical, and Gynecological Complications of Pregnancy. Williams and Wilkins, Baltimore, 1965.
7. Garry J: Abdominal surgery during pregnancy. Obstet Gynecol 10:660, 1951.
8. Shnider SM, Webster GM: Maternal and fetal hazards of surgery during pregnancy. Am J Obstet Gynecol 92:891, 1965.
9. Cavanagh D: Surgical emergencies in obstetrics. p. 375–396. In Cavanagh D, Ed: Obstetrical Emergencies. Harper & Row, Hagerstown, 1978.

10. Baer JR, Reis RA, Arens RA: Appendicitis in pregnancy. Obstet Gynecol 46:655–662, 1975.
11. Hoffman ES, Suzuki M: Acute appendicitis in pregnancy; ten year survey. Am J Obstet Gynecol 67:1338, 1954.
12. Chamberlain G: Gynaecological aspects of the acute abdomen. Ann RC Surg 45:174–185, 1969.
13. Benson CD: Surgical implications of Meckel's diverticulitis. In Mustard WT, et al, Eds: Pediatric Surgery. Vol. 2. p. 864. Yearbook Medical Publishers, Chicago, 1969.
14. Lindheimer MD, Katz AI: Kidney Function and Disease in Pregnancy. Lea and Febiger, Philadelphia, 1977, p. 108.
15. Kass EH, Savage A, Santamarina BA: The significance of bacteriuria in preventive medicine. In Kass EH, Ed: Progress in Pyelonephritis. p. 3. F. A. Davis, Philadelphia, 1965.
16. Harris RE: Obstetrical urinary tract infection. USAF MC Lackland AFB, TX.
17. Harris RE, Dunnihoo DR: The incidence and significance of urinary calculi in pregnancy. Am J Obstet Gynecol 97:720, 1967.
18. Folger GK: Pain and pregnancy; treatment of painful states complicating pregnancy, with particular emphasis on urinary calculi. Obstet Gynecol 5:513–518, 1955.
19. Coe FL, Parks JH, Lindheimer MD: Nephrolithiasis during pregnancy. N Engl J Med 298:324–326, 1978.
20. Hill LM, Johnson CE, Lee RA: Ovarian surgery in pregnancy. Am J Obstet Gynecol 122:565–569, 1975.
21. Booth RT: Ovarian tumors in pregnancy. Obstet Gynecol 21:189–193, 1963.
22. Pritchard JA, Macdonald PC: Dystocia caused by other abnormalities of the reproductive tract. In: Williams Obstetrics. 15th Ed. p. 719. Appleton-Century-Crofts, New York, 1976.
23. Corlett RG, Mishell DR: Pancreatitis in pregnancy. Am J Obstet Gynecol 13:281–290, 1972.
24. Jouppila P, Mokka R, Larmi TK: Acute pancreatitis in pregnancy. Surg Gynecol Obstet 139:879–882, 1974.
25. Buchsbaum HJ: Trauma in Pregnancy. W. B. Saunders, Philadelphia, 1979.
26. Cruikshank DP: Anatomic and physiologic alterations of pregnancy that modify the response to trauma. In: Trauma in Pregnancy. W. B. Saunders, Philadelphia, 1979.
27. Peckman CH, King RW: A study of intercurrent conditions observed during pregnancy. Am J Obstet Gynecol 87:609, 1963.
28. Buchsbaum HJ: Accidental injury complicating pregnancy. Am J Obstet Gynecol 102:752, 1968.

4 Hypertensive Disorders of Pregnancy

Ralph T. DePalma

In the early twentieth century maternal mortality from eclampsia approached 30 percent.[1] Since World War II results have improved. As recently as 1967, though, 10.3 percent of 107 women with eclampsia in one series died, despite treatment with chorpromazine, diethazine, and meperidine.[2] At Parkland Memorial Hospital in Dallas, Texas, more than 170 women have been treated consecutively since 1955 for eclampsia, with one maternal death.[3,4] Because of the severe consequences associated with eclampsia, hypertension is always treated as an emergency. All women are hospitalized once the diagnosis is suspected.

The emergency room physician, who initiates the treatment of the pregnant hypertensive patient, has as his main objective the prevention or control of eclampsia and its devastating consequences. This goal may be achieved by lowering dangerously elevated blood pressures and by preventing or suppressing seizure activity. Therefore, in the acute emergency room situation, hypertension, regardless of its etiology, is treated in a standard manner, utilizing magnesium sulfate and hydralazine as outlined later in this chapter. If this simple method for treating acute hypertension in pregnancy is followed, both maternal and fetal mortality and morbidity will be kept to a minimum.

Hypertension may be classified by many different schemes, but for the purpose of this chapter, three categories are considered: eclampsia; preeclampsia or pregnancy-induced hypertension; and chronic hypertension, with or without pregnancy-induced hypertension. Eclampsia is considered first because of its morbid sequelae. A brief discussion of the underlying pathophysiology of hypertension is included in the section devoted to preeclampsia and chronic hypertension.

ECLAMPSIA

Eclampsia is the most severe manifestation of hypertension during pregnancy. This acute disorder is characterized by clonic and tonic convulsions that in some way are caused by hypertension, induced or aggravated by pregnancy. Clinically, the disease manifests itself most often during the third trimester, with increasing frequency as term approaches. Invariably, preeclampsia precedes the onset of convulsions; however, seizures may occur with mild hypertension in the absence of proteinuria.

The convulsions usually begin as a facial twitch. Rapidly the entire body becomes rigid with generalized muscle contractions. The violent force of the contraction may cause physical injury to the patient. After the convulsion, coma ensues. The process may repeat itself numerous times in untreated cases. Along with blood pressure, respirations are increased, presumably in response to hypercarbia from lactic acidemia. Severe hyperthermia (103°F) is rare. It is believed to be central in origin and carries a poor prognosis. Massive cerebral hemorrhage may cause sudden death. Pulmonary edema from congestive heart failure, aspiration of gastric contents, cyanosis, rising tachycardia, and worsening hypotension are common in fatal cases only. If the patient does not immediately succumb following aspiration, bronchopneumonia often develops. Subcapsular hemorrhage in the liver may rupture, resulting in death from massive bleeding into the peritoneal cavity. Proteinuria is almost always present and is often pronounced. Urine output is usually decreased and at times ceases altogether. Renal cortical necrosis may supervene with gradually worsening azotemia and death. Edema, at times anasarca, is usually seen. Occasionally blindness from retinal edema occurs; however, retinal detachment is rare. Psychosis following eclampsia usually carries a good prognosis except when there is pre-existing mental illness. Indeed, eclampsia may be devastating to both mother and fetus if treatment is not quickly and vigorously instituted.

Treatment of eclampsia at Parkland Memorial Hospital [5] has been standardized since 1955 and consists of (1) intravenous and intramuscular magnesium sulfate ($MgSO_4.7H_2O$ USP) to arrest convulsions and prevent their recurrence; (2) intravenous hydralazine intermittently to control diastolic blood pressures in excess of 110 mm Hg; and (3) delivery of the patient once her condition stabilizes. To control an eclamptic seizure, $MgSO_4.7H_2O$ USP, 4 g intravenously (20 percent solution when given IV),* is given over 3 minutes, followed by 10 g $MgSO_4.7H_2O$ USP (50 percent solution with 1 cc of 1 percent lidocaine) intramuscularly (5 g in each buttock), followed by 5 g intramuscularly every 4 hours if the respiratory rate is not depressed, patellar reflexes are present, and urinary output has been at least 100 cc or more in the previous 4 hours. If seizure activity recurs, an additional 2 to 4 g of intravenous $MgSO_4.7H_2O$ USP may be given (Table 4.1).

---

* 20 ml of 20 percent magnesium sulfate can be made by mixing 8 ml of50 percent magnesium sulfate solution with 12 ml of sterile water.

Table 4-1. Treatment of Hypertensive Crisis in Pregnancy.

1. $MgSO_4$—20% solution—4 g IV
2. $MgSO_4$—50% solution—10 g IM then 5 g IM q4h
3. Hydralazine—5–10 mg IM q 10–20 mins until diastolic approximately 100 mm Hg
4. $MgSO_4$—20% solution—2–4 g IV with recurrent seizures
5. Maintain airway
6. Prevent injury with padded restraints
7. Monitor urinary output
8. Monitor CVP
9. Delivery of fetus when patient is stabilized

Care must be taken to protect the eclamptic patient from injuring herself. A padded tongue blade will minimize trauma to the tongue. Firm but gentle restraint will prevent fractures of the long bones or vertebrae. The patient's head should be lowered, the oropharynx suctioned, an airway established, and oxygen administered. The last steps will help prevent aspiration and its grim consequences. Sodium amobarbital and sodium thiopental are avoided initially because they produce sedation. There is also evidence that these anticonvulsants decrease cerebral oxygenation while $MgSO_4.7H_2O$ USP does not.[6] If $MgSO_4.7H_2O$ USP fails to control convulsions, then sodlum amobarbital, 250 mg intravenously, may be administered slowly, over no less than 3 minutes. Valium has been advocated for the control of eclampsia, and while it may be effective in the control of seizures, at Parkland Memorial Hospital diazepam is not used because of the profound depressant effects exerted on both mother and fetus.[7] Every pregnant woman has the potential for aspiration of gastric contents, and Valium, as well as other sedative anticonvulsants, will serve only to increase the risk of this dangerous complication. Moreover, resuscitation in the newborn infant is far more difficult after diazepam administration to the mother, because respiratory depression and hypotonicity are caused by this drug and are not reversible.

Antihypertensive therapy for eclampsia is given only if diastolic blood pressure exceeds 110 mm Hg.[8] Any attempts to lower the blood pressure below a range of 90 to 100 mm Hg may compromise uteroplacental perfusion and result in further fetal jeopardy. Hydralazine, 5 mg intravenously every 10 to 20 minutes, is given to accomplish this. The dose of hydralazine may be increased by 5 to 10 mg if necessary. A total dose of 5 to 20 mg of apresoline is usually sufficient. Hydralazine is the only antihypertensive drug which does not decrease uteroplacental blood flow in the experimental animal.[9] Recently, diazoxide [10,11] has been recommended to control dangerously high blood pressures during pregnancy. Diazoxide exerts its effects by direct relaxation of arteriolar smooth muscle in all vascular beds.[12] Unlike hydralazine, however, diazoxide decreases uterine blood flow [9,13] and hence is potentially dangerous to the fetus. The use of methyldopa, reserpine, guanethidine, and thiazide diuretics is advocated by some [10,14,15] for "chronic" treatment of hypertension in pregnancy, but they have no role in the acute management of this problem.

Urinary output is monitored hourly. Oliguria or anuria reflects the underlying intense vasospasm, hypovolemia from blood loss, or both. Diuretics should, therefore, be avoided, unless pulmonary edema develops; then furosemide is the drug of choice. Mannitol, hypertonic dextrose, and albumin are never used at Parkland Memorial Hospital in an attempt to mobilize extravascular fluid or increase urinary output. Lactated Ringer's solution is infused at a rate of 60 to 125 cc per hour. Whole blood is given for excessive blood loss. In the eclamptic patient, administration of fluids may best be accomplished while monitoring central venous pressure in addition to urine output. In this way, pulmonary edema may be avoided. Laboratory studies may be kept to a minimum. Hematocrit, urinalysis, serum creatinine and electrolytes, leukocyte and platelet counts, and careful examination of plasma for abnormal amounts of heme pigments should be done. Whole blood should be readily available if hemorrhage becomes excessive.

Delivery is attempted only after the patient's condition is stable. Fetal bradycardia after a convulsion is most likely a consequence of acidosis and hypoxia induced by intense muscular contractions, and is not an indication for immediate cesarean section. Treatment of the mother's hypoxia and convulsions will likely improve the condition of the fetus as well. Induction with oxytocin may be tried if there is no obstetric contraindication to vaginal delivery; otherwise, cesarean section is performed.

Using this approach for the treatment of eclampsia, Pritchard had one maternal death in the last 25 years, and his perinatal mortality rate was 15.9 percent, including 12 fetuses weighting less than 1,000 g.[3,4]

PREECLAMPSIA (PREGNANCY-INDUCED HYPERTENSION) AND CHRONIC HYPERTENSION WITH SUPERIMPOSED PREECLAMPSIA

Whether the woman has "pure" preeclampsia or chronic hypertension with superimposed preeclampsia, the treatment regimens are identical and include prevention of convulsions and control of dangerously high blood pressures. Chronic hypertension without superimposed preeclampsia is treated differently and will be considered separately. In order to understand the treatment of hypertension, the physician must first understand some of the normal physiologic changes and then the aberrant changes specifically related to pregnancy-induced hypertension (PIH).

During pregnancy blood volume increases as much as 50 percent.[16] This increase is due mainly to plasma volume alterations, but during the third trimester red blood cell volume increases as well. Cardiac output is also elevated by as much as 50 percent.[17] This change in cardiac output is mainly due to an increase in stroke volume secondary to increased venous return to the right heart. An increase in heart rate contributes also but to a lesser degree. Despite this, blood pressure, especially during the second trimester, is significantly lower.[18] This can be explained entirely by a marked drop in the total peripheral resistance, which is probably an effect of progesterone.[19]

In contrast, blood volume in a pregnancy complicated by preeclampsia is relatively decreased as a combined result of vasospasm and fluid loss to extravascular spaces.[20] Cardiac output, however, usually does not decrease and may remain unchanged.[17,21] The widespread intermittent vasospasm characteristic of preeclampsia causes peripheral resistance to increase dramatically, resulting in the elevated blood pressure. Vascular sensitivity to angiotensin II is markedly elevated in these women.[18] This alteration in response to angiotensin may cause increased vasospasm, further compounding the hypertension and diminished intravascular volume. These changes are responsible for the decrease in renal blood flow during the hypertensive pregnancy.[22]

In addition to the decrease or absence of pregnancy hypervolemia in most hypertensive patients, occasional alterations of the coagulation mechanism and hemolysis may occur. These changes are directly related to the severity and duration of the disease process but are most certainly not causes of the hypertension itself.[23]

Clinically, certain problems arise as a result of the changes initiated by hypertension. Because of the contracted intravascular volume, fluid administration, if not done carefully, frequently causes volume overload with pulmonary edema. In most hypertensive situations in pregnancy, diuretics are contraindicated because they further decrease the already compromised intravascular volume. Congestive heart failure with pulmonary edema is the only condition in which these drugs are appropriate.

At the opposite end of the spectrum, blood loss is often tolerated poorly by the hypertensive gravida, because of the aforementioned reduction in blood volume. An immediate amelioration in hypertension following delivery must be viewed with extreme suspicion. This situation suggests excessive blood loss requiring transfusion, rather than relief of the underlying vasospasm following pregnancy termination. Oliguria less than 30 cc per hour must also be considered a result of blood loss. Treatment with transfusions and balanced salt solutions, rather than diuretics, should be considered. Diuretics will serve only to contract further the decreased blood volume and must be avoided when oliguria is present.

In severe preeclampsia or eclampsia, evidence of a mircroangiopathic hemolytic anemia may be present.[23] This is a consequence of the severe vasospasm and a resultant adhesion of fibrin strands to structurally altered endothelial surfaces. The red blood cell (RBC) membranes are damaged as they traverse these small blood vessels, thus leading to hemolysis. This hemolytic anemia rarely presents a problem because it is rapidly reversed with delivery of the patient and ultimate relief of the vasospasm. Treatment, therefore, is the safe, expeditious delivery of the patient. Occasionally, thrombocytopenia and anemia are severe enough to warrant platelet packs or packed red blood cells. If hemorrhage occurs, transfusion with whole blood may be necessary. Heparin under these circumstances is absolutely contraindicated because it will worsen hemorrhage and, in the hypertensive patient, predispose to intracranial bleeding.

Coagulopathy, or disseminated intravascular coagulation, (DIC), as a result of PIH, seldom occurs. Hence its clinical significance is minimal. Pritchard and coworkers [23] have shown that only a small minority of patients with severe preeclampsia/eclampsia demonstrate the thrombocytopenia associated with microangiopathic hemolysis. Even fewer patients with eclampsia show decreased plasma fibrinogen or the presence of fibrin split products. Hence a cause and effect relationship between DIC and preeclampsia/eclampsia remains to be shown. While the thrombocytopenia associated with microangiopathic hemolysis seems to correlate with the severity of the hypertension in pregnancy, plasma fibrinogen and fibrin degradation products do not.

The physician must always consider the effects of drug administration in the unborn child. In order to understand the rationale for treating the pregnant hypertensive patient in such a way that adverse fetal consequences are avoided, the physiology of both the maternal and fetoplacental units must be reviewed. MacDonald and Siiteri [24] have shown that one-half of the estradiol (E2) produced by the placenta is derived from maternal dehydroepiandrosterone sulfate (DS). Everett, et al [25] have shown that the placental clearance of DS to E2 reflects uteroplacental blood flow. Utilizing this information, Gant, et al [26–31] demonstrated that the metabolic clearance, as well as the placental clearance (PC), of DS to E2 in pregnancies complicated by preeclampsia is higher than clearances in normal pregnancies, starting as early as the 22nd week of gestation. These clearances, however, begin to decrease approximately 3 to 4 weeks prior to the onset of overt hypertension. Those patients with chronic hypertension destined to develop superimposed preeclampsia demonstrate this same phenomenon. Shoemaker, et al [32] have measured PCDS-E2 in patients on thiazide diuretics and have shown a significant decrease in clearances among all women tested. Therefore, it is presumed that any treatment which further alters uteroplacental blood flow may be devastating to an already compromised fetus.

At Parkland Memorial Hospital, treatment of hypertension, either preeclampsia or chronic with superimposed preeclampsia, is given to insure maximum benefit to both mother and fetus. If the diastolic blood pressure exceeds 90 mm Hg, the patient is hospitalized. Whalley has shown that the perinatal mortality rate for patients with PIH who were hospitalized early is 9/1,000.[33] This contrasts with a perinatal mortality rate of 129/1,000 among those who refused admission.[33] Once the patient is hospitalized, management begins with questions pertaining to visual disturbances, headaches, epigastric or right upper quadrant pain, and uterine pain or bleeding. If these symptoms of severe preeclampsia are present, medication to prevent convulsions is immediately indicated. The physical examination should include an assessment of the optic fundi for signs of chronic hypertensive disease and/or preeclampsia. A search must be instituted for evidence of cardiovascular compromise, i.e., pulmonary edema from congestive heart failure. Evaluation for liver or uterine tenderness will give clues to possible hemorrhage into the liver capsule or hemorrhage from a placental abruption. An evaluation of the uterine cervix is helpful in rationally planning for delivery. Detection of clonus in the deep tendon reflexes may indicate imminent eclampsia.

Initial treatment for severe preeclampsia—blood pressure greater than 160 mm Hg systolic or 110 mm Hg diastolic, 3 or 4 plus proteinuria on qualitative examination, central or visual disturbances, epigastric pain, pulmonary edema or cyanosis—requires an intravenous line for the administering of medication to prevent or control convulsions, the lowering of blood pressure, and the administering of fluids for replacement of insensible water loss, urine output, or excessive blood loss at delivery.

Magnesium sulfate is the treatment of choice for both prevention and control of convulsions in the hypertensive patient.[4,34] To prevent seizure activity, the patient is treated with a loading dose of 10 g of $MgSO_4.7H_2O$ USP (a 50 percent solution with 1 cc 1 percent lidocaine) intramuscularly (5 g in each buttock) followed by 5 g intramuscularly every 4 hours as outlined in the section on eclampsia. If administered in this manner, magnesium sulfate is extremely safe and effective. If impending eclampsia is suspected because of severe headache, scotomata, epigastric or right upper quadrant pain, or ankle clonus, intravenous magnesium sulfate is given initially and followed by the intramuscular dose as outlined above. Usually 2 g of intravenous $MgSO_4.7H_2O$ USP (20 percent solution when given IV) is sufficient for this purpose. Antihypertensive therapy is administered in the manner described for eclampsia.

CHRONIC HYPERTENSION WITHOUT SUPERIMPOSED PREECLAMPSIA

Women with chronic hypertension are hospitalized at Parkland Memorial Hospital if diastolic blood pressures exceed 90 mm Hg. They are then treated expectantly, avoiding antihypertensive medications except in certain rigidly defined circumstances. Prior to 20 weeks gestation, diuretics may be given if diastolic blood pressures are consistently above 90 mm Hg. During the second half of pregnancy, diuretics are avoided because of the adverse effects they exert on uterine blood flow. Methyldopa, apresoline, and propranolol, in that order, have been used with some success in the treatment of chronic hypertension at Parkland Memorial Hospital. If diastolic blood pressure exceeds 100 mm Hg, these agents are given to lower blood pressure to a range of 90 to 100 mm Hg. However, chronic antihypertensive medication is rarely needed because most patients respond to hospitalization alone. In addition, the pregnancy associated reduction in blood pressure during the second trimester aids in maintaining blood pressure in an acceptable range.

The efforts of the physician in the management of the hypertensive gravida are directed toward the delivery of a robust, mature infant to a healthy mother. Avoidance of severe hypertension and convulsions is the main objective in the management of these women. Effective and judicious use of hospitalization, magnesium sulfate, and hydralazine will usually lead to a good outcome in most patients.

REFERENCES

1. Holland E: The results of a collective investigation into cesarean sections performed in Great Britain and Ireland from the year 1911 to 1920 inclusive. Br J Obstet Gynaecol 28:358, 1921.
2. Lopez-Llera M: Eclampsia 1963–1966. Evaluation of the treatment of 107 cases. Br J Obstet Gynaecol 74:379, 1967.
3. Pritchard JA: Personal communication.
4. Pritchard JA, Pritchard SA: Standardized treatment of 154 consecutive cases of eclampsia. Am J Obstet Gynecol 123:543, 1975.
5. Pritchard JA, MacDonald PC: Eclampsia treatment at Parkland Memorial Hospital. p. 572. In Williams Obstetrics. 15th Ed. Appleton-Century-Crofts, New York, 1976.
6. McCall ML, Sass D: The action of magnesium sulfate on cerebral circulation and metabolism in toxemia of pregnancy. Am J Obstet Gynecol 71:1089, 1956.
7. Gant NF, Worley RJ: Prevention of convulsions. p. 115. In Hypertension in Pregnancy: Concepts and Management. Appleton-Century-Crofts, New York, 1980.
8. Feitelson PJ, Lindheimer MD: Management of hypertensive gravidas. J Reprod Med 8:111, 1972.
9. Brinkman III CR, Assali NS: Uteroplacental hemodynamic response to antihypertensive drugs in hypertensive pregnant sheep. In Lindheimer MD, Katz AI, Zuspan FP, Eds: Hypertension in Pregnancy. Wiley, New York, 1976.
10. Finnerty Jr FA: Hypertensive emergencies. In Laragh JH, Ed: Hypertension Manual: Mechanisms, Methods, Management. York, New York, 1974.
11. Pennington JC, Picker RH: Diazoxide and the treatment of the acute hypertensive emergency in obstetrics. Med J Aust 2:1051, 1972.
12. Koch-Weser, J: Diazoxide. N Eng J Med 294:1271, 1976.
13. Caritas SN, Morishima HO, Stark RI, James LS: The effect of diazoxide on uterine blood flow in pregnant sheep. Obstet Gynecol 48:464, 1976.
14. Ferris TF: Toxemia and hypertension. In Burrow GN, Ferris TF, Eds: Medical Complications During Pregnancy. W.B. Saunders, Philadelphia, 1975.
15. Ferris TF: Hypertension in pregnancy. Perinat Care 2:4, 1978.
16. Pritchard JA: Changes in blood volume during pregnancy and delivery. Anesthesia 26:393, 1965.
17. Werko L: Studies in the problems of circulation in pregnancy. p. 155. In Hammond J, Crowne FJ, Wolstenholm GEW, Eds: Toxemias of Pregnancy: Human and Veterinary. Blakeston, Philadelphia, 1950.
18. Gant NF, Daley GL, Chand S, et al: A study of angiotensin II pressor response throughout primigravid pregnancy. J Clin Invest 52:2682, 1973.
19. Gant NF, Worley RJ: Cardiac output. p. 42. In Hypertension in Pregnancy: Concepts and Management. Appleton-Century-Crofts, New York, 1980.
20. Gant NF, Worley RJ: Blood volume changes. p. 44. In Hypertension in Pregnancy: Concepts and Management. Appleton-Century-Crofts, New York, 1980.
21. Assali NS, Holm LW, Parker HR: Systemic and regional hemodynamic alterations in toxemia. Circulation 30(S2):53, 1964.

22. Chesley LC, Duffus GM: Preeclampsia, posture, and renal function. Obstet Gynecol 38:1, 1971.
23. Pritchard JA, Cunningham FG, Mason RA: Coagulation changes in eclampsia: their frequency and pathogenesis. Am J Obstet Gynecol 124:855, 1976.
24. Siiteri PK, MacDonald PC: The utilization of circulating dehydroisoandrosterone sulfate for estrogen synthesis during human pregnancy. Steroids 2:713, 1963.
25. Everett RB, Gant NF, Porter JC, MacDonald PC: Relationship of placental blood flow to the placental clearance of maternal plasma dehydroisoandrosterone sulfate (DS) through estradiol (PC-DSE2). Proceedings of the Society for Gynecologic Investigation, March 1978 (Abstract).
26. Gant NF, Hutchinson HT, Siiteri PK, MacDonald PC: Study of the metabolic clearance rate of dehydroisoandrosterone sulfate in pregnancy. Am J Obstet Gynecol 111:555, 1971.
27. Gant NF, Madden JD, Chand S, et al: Metabolic clearance rate of dehydroisoandrosterone sulfate. V. Studies of essential hypertension complicating pregnancy. Obstet Gynecol 47:319, 1976.
28. Gant NF, Madden JD, Chand S, et al: Metabolic clearance rate of dehydroisoandrosterone sulfate. VI. Studies of eclampsia. Obstet Gynecol 47:327, 1976.
29. Gant NF, Madden JD, Siiteri PK, MacDonald PC: A sequential study of the metabolism of dehydroisoandrosterone sulfate in primigravid pregnancy. Proceedings of the Fourth International Congress of Endocrinology. Amsterdam, Excerpta Medica, 1972, p. 1096 (Abstract).
30. Gant NF, Madden JD, Siiteri PK, MacDonald PC: The metabolic clearance rate of dehydroisoandrosterone sulfate. III. The effect of thiazide diuretics in normal and future preeclamptic pregnancies. Am J Obstet Gynecol 123:159, 1975.
31. Gant NF, Madden JD, Siiteri PK, MacDonald PC: The metabolic clearance rate of dehydroisoandrosterone sulfate. IV. Acute effects of induced hypertension, hypotension, and naturesis in normal and hypertensive pregnancies. Am J Obstet Gynecol 124:143, 1976.
32. Shoemaker ES, Gant NF, Madden JD, MacDonald PC: The effect of thiazide diuretics on placental function. Tex Med 69:109, 1973.
33. Gilstrap LC, Cunningham FG, Whalley PJ: Management of pregnancy-induced hypertension in the nulliparous patient remote from term. Semin Perinatol 2:73, 1978.
34. Pritchard JA: Management of severe preeclampsia and eclampsia. Semin Perinatol 2:83, 1978.

5 Acute Medical Emergencies in Obstetrics

Arnold W. Cohen

Obstetrical emergencies tax the knowledge and expertise of any physician called upon to care for the patient. Medical decisions have to be made which not only insure the health of the mother, the primary patient, but maximize the safety of the fetus. Whatever the acute medical emergency may be, the emergency room physician may be the first doctor called upon to evaluate and treat the pregnant patient. Because of this, it behooves any physician who works in an emergency room to understand (1) the unique physiologic changes that occur during pregnancy, (2) the effect that the medical disease has on the mother and fetus, and (3) what effect any treatment given to the mother will have on the fetus. Underlying any therapeutic decision made during pregnancy has to be the realization that maternal well-being must be guarded and maintained. At times, a problem arises where acute treatment of the mother may compromise the safety of the fetus; i.e., cardiac by-pass used in open heart surgery. I believe maternal considerations should be primary in the treating physician's thoughts. Once an appropriate course of therapy is determined, then modifications should be made to minimize dangers to the fetus. When this approach is taken, the physician has fulfilled his obligation to the mother and her unborn child.

Other chapters cover acute obstetrical and gynecologic emergencies. This chapter focuses on some common medical problems which occur during pregnancy, and stresses: (1) the physiologic principles which make treatment of a pregnant patient different from treatment of the non-pregnant patient, (2) fetal considerations, and (3) a simplified treatment plan that can be initiated by the emergency room physician, prior to the availability of the obstetrician, who should have primary responsibility for the health and well-being of both the mother and the fetus.

DIABETIC KETOACIDOSIS

Pregnancy causes a decrease in serum glucose and amino acids. This is because of a continuous "siphoning off" of these molecules by the fetus, and changes in placental hormones as the pregnancy progresses. Because of these metabolic changes, there is an increased utilization of lipids, resulting in increased ketone bodies and free fatty acids. By 15 weeks of gestation, there is a noticeable early morning hypoglycemia that increases the normally occurring ketone body formation after an overnight fast. Serum beta-hydroxybutyric acids and acetoacetate acids are 2 to 4 times higher after an overnight fast in a pregnant patient than in the non-pregnant patient.[1] Hyperketonuria results in increased ketone bodies in amniotic fluid. The fetus can use this metabolic fuel in the face of decreased glucose supplies. Fetal brain tissue has the enzymes necessary to utilize ketone bodies,[2] but whether the use of this fuel promotes optimum fetal brain growth is questioned.[3]

The hormonal changes during pregnancy exert a contrainsulin effect. Human placental lactogen (HPL) is the major placental hormone produced by the syncytiotrophoblast that counteracts the action of insulin. Increases in estrogen, progesterone, free cortisol, and growth hormone also contribute to the anti-insulin effect of pregnancy. These hormonal changes necessitate increased insulin release from the normal pancreas during pregnancy, or an increase in exogenous insulin needs in the insulin-dependent diabetic. The hormonal changes are such that insulin requirements stay stable, or actually decrease somewhat, during the first trimester. They then rise to 100 to 400 percent above pre-pregnancy doses. Because of this increased insulin requirement, as well as the lipolytic effect of HPL, acetonuria and ketonemia occur easily during pregnancy.

When ketoacidosis occurs during pregnancy, the incidence of fetal deaths may approach or surpass 50 percent.[4] Before any treatment is initiated though, starvation ketosis must be distinguished from diabetic ketoacidosis. Overnight fasting, nausea, vomiting, and restricted caloric intake can cause acetonuria and even increases in serum ketoacids. These two conditions can be differentiated by testing the urine for glucosuria or getting a serum glucose value. If the urine dipstick is negative for glucose, or if the blood sugar is less than 150 mg/dl, then starvation ketosis is more likely than diabetic ketoacidosis. This patient should be treated with glucose solutions and not insulin.

When diabetic ketoacidosis is present, adequate treatment of the initiating cause, as well as fluids, insulin, bicarbonate, and potassium, will usually avoid a maternal mortality but will not assure the health of the fetus. Many times when the patient presents in ketoacidosis, an intrauterine demise has already occurred. Whatever the status of the fetus on admission, correction of maternal acidemia, dehydration, and hypokalemia should be accomplished before any steps are taken to deliver the fetus.

The hormonal changes previously noted may promote ketosis, but ketoacidosis occurs only when there is a relative or absolute deficiency of insulin. This most commonly occurs when the patient forgets to take her insulin, but other initiating events should be sought after. The patient should be evaluated for a superimposed infection: either pneumonia, upper respiratory infection (URI), or pyelonephritis. An increase in steroid dosage during the pregnancy, or steroids acutely administered, may cause a relative insulin deficiency and precipitate ketoacidosis. Other initiating events as hyperthyroidism, hypokalemia, and diuretic or thyroid therapy are rarely found in pregnant patients. When the initiating event for ketoacidosis is found, it should be treated aggressively. If no initiating event is found, the patient should be re-evaluated for these factors after the acute episode is successfully treated (Table 5.1).

Pathophysiologic changes of diabetic ketoacidosis must be understood to effect appropriate therapy. Insulin deficiency produces an increase in hepatic gluconeogenesis, but a decrease in peripheral glucose utilization. The resulting hyperglycemia produces an osmotic diuresis which causes severe dehydration. Lack of adequate insulin also produces increased fatty acid release from adipose tissue, an increased hepatic ketone production, and a decrease in peripheral utilization of ketone bodies. These changes result in ketonemia and acidosis. Successful therapy of diabetic ketoacidosis in the pregnant, as well as non-pregnant, patient requires effective doses of insulin, as well as correction of intracellular and extracellular fluids and electrolytes. The patient should be followed frequently with blood pressure measurements, pulse, mental status evaluation, input and output determinations. Laboratory determination of blood glucose, ketones, potassium, sodium, bicarbonate, blood urea nitrogen (BUN), creatinine, and phosphate should be done on admission. Baseline arterial blood gases, pH, and electrocardiogram should be obtained. If there is any evidence of pulmonary infection or any auscultatory findings on the chest examination, a chest x-ray should be done with adequate shielding of the uterus. Plasma electrolytes, glucose, and arterial blood gases should be repeated every 1 to 2 hours, depending on the clinical state of the patient.

Insulin therapy should be initiated as soon as the diagnosis is established. Controversy exists among advocates of continuous intravenous, intramuscular, and subcutaneous administration techniques. Low dose insulin therapy is as effective in normalizing plasma glucose, bicarbonate, ketone bodies, and blood

Table 5-1. Precipitating causes of ketoacidosis.

1. Patient neglect
2. Infection—pneumonia, pyelonephritis, URI
3. Steroid therapy
4. Hyperthyroidism
5. Hypokalemia
6. Diuretics
7. Thyroid medications

pH as high dose IV and subcutaneous therapy.[5] Besides the ease of therapy with low dose insulin, there is less hypoglycemia and hypokalemia associated with this form.

Low dose insulin therapy for ketoacidosis can be accomplished by IV continuous infusion or by intermittent intramuscular injections. Continuous intravenous insulin therapy is initiated with 0.15 units/Kg body weight (8 to 14 units), and is followed by 7 to 10 units/hr in normal saline. If the blood glucose has not fallen by 75 to 100 mg/dl during the first 2 hours of therapy, the infusion rate should be increased to 15 to 20 units/hr. When the plasma glucose has reached 250 mg/dl, glucose is given in the IV solution in order to minimize the chance of severe hypoglycemia. The IV insulin infusion is continued until the pH normalizes and blood sugar values return to 150 to 250 mg/dl. If IM insulin is to be used, the patient is given 10 to 15 units. This is followed by 5 to 10 units IM every 1 hr when blood sugar values are obtainable rapidly, or 10 to 15 units IM every 2 hours if lab results are not immediately available. When the blood glucose reaches 250 mg/dl, glucose is added to the IV solution, as is done when IV insulin is used. With both regimens, when the patient's glucose and pH are stabilized, she should be treated with regular insulin given subcutaneously every 4 hours. The next day she can be given her normal dose of long and short acting insulins.

Successful treatment of diabetic ketoacidosis does not depend only on adequate insulin therapy. Correction of fluid and electrolyte abnormalities may require the administration of 2 to 3 liters of Ringer's Lactate or 0.45 percent sodium chloride solution supplemented with 45 meq of sodium bicarbonate (1 ampule). Additional sodium bicarbonate therapy should be given only if the patient's initial pH is less than 7.1, or the pH is less than 7.2 and the patient is hypotensive, or in a coma. In patients who are hypotensive, 0.9 percent sodium chloride solution plus albumin may be used as initial therapy. If the patient's blood pressure, urine output, and vital signs do not improve rapidly, a central venous pressure (CVP) line should be inserted. After the first several liters of fluid are given, 2 to 3 liters more should be given over the next 24 hours as 0.45 percent sodium chloride, or D5W and 0.45 percent sodium chloride when the plasma glucose falls to 250 mg/dl.

Diabetic ketoacidosis is associated with a total body loss of 5 to 10 meq/Kg body weight of potassium. Because of this, patients with a normal serum potassium should have 40 meq of $K+$ added to the first liter of solution and 20 to 40 meq to each subsequent bottle. If the initial $K+$ is elevated, potassium should be added when the plasma glucose and $K+$ start to fall, usually with the second liter of solution.

Phosphate depletion also occurs with diabetic ketoacidosis. This affects erythrocyte 2, 3 DPG so that the oxygen dissociation curve is shifted to the left. This causes a decreased ability of the red blood cells to deliver O_2 to the tissues, with resulting tissue and cerebral hypoxia. Its affects on the fetus have never been evaluated in human diabetics in ketoacidosis, but may be one of the reasons there is such a high perinatal mortality rate associated with this condition. To correct the phosphate depletion, IV potassium phosphate, 2.5 to 5.0 meq/Kg body weight over 6 to 8 hours, or Phospho-Soda, 5 ml orally tid, is given. Serum phosphate and calcium should be monitored daily (Table 5.2).

If the patient admitted with diabetic ketoacidosis has no fetal heart tones audible, Dopler instruments should be used to ascertain the viability of the fetus. If an intrauterine demise has occurred and is confirmed by real-time ultrasonography, the mother should be stabilized. Only after several days of control should a decision be made to terminate the pregnancy with prostaglandin E_2 suppositories or to allow the pregnancy to continue until there is the spontaneous onset of labor. I favor termination of the pregnancy soon after an intrauterine fetal demise has been diagnosed and the patient stabilized, because the rapid changes in the placental contrainsulin hormones will make control of the diabetes difficult. Even in a patient with a very unfavorable cervix, prostaglandins will effect delivery within 12 to 48 hours. During that time, the patient is maintained NPO with 10 units of insulin in each bottle of D5½ NS given at 125 cc/hr. Plasma glucose determinations should be done every 2 to 4 hours and the infusion rate adjusted accordingly.

When fetal viability is established in a patient over 28 weeks of gestation, the patient should have continuous fetal heart monitoring. If evidence of fetal distress occurs, the mother can be given oxygen and put in the left lateral decubitus position. If these maneuvers do not alleviate the fetal distress, then the physician must determine if immediate delivery is necessary for fetal survival. If the mother's condition is still unstable, no intervention on behalf of the fetus is indicated.

Once the pregnant patient with diabetic ketoacidosis has recovered, a decision must be made as to where the patient can best be treated for the remainder of the pregnancy. If the inciting cause has been identified and treated, the patient may be sent home on her usual dosage of insulin. If no inciting cause can be found, the patient should be hospitalized for an extended period of time so that she can be placed on appropriate dosages of insulin, be instructed in proper diet, and learn to use a glucose reflectance meter. These measures will allow her to maintain her plasma glucose levels in good control for the remainder of her pregnancy and maximize the chance of a good outcome for both the mother and the fetus.

Table 5-2. Treatment of diabetic-ketoacidosis.

1. Treat initiating cause
2. Baseline laboratory values—Glucose, Serum Ketones, K+, CO_2, BUN, Creatinine, PO_4, ABG, ECG, CXR
3. Insulin Therapy
   a. IV Therapy—0.15 units/Kg then 7–10 units/hr
   b. IM Therapy—10–15 units then 5–10 units q 1 hr
4. Fluids—Ringer's Lactate or 0.9% NaCl: 2–3 liters rapidly then 150–200 cc/hr. When Blood Sugar is <250 mg/dl use D5NS and add K+ 40 MEg./l to solution.
5. Potassium phosphate—2.5–5.0 mg/Kg q 8 hr
6. Regular insulin—SC q 4 hr × 24 hr after initial stabilization
7. Usual dose of NPH & regular

PULMONARY EDEMA

Cardiac disease occurs in 1 to 2 percent of all pregnancies.[6] Rheumatic heart disease, specifically mitral stenosis, still accounts for the majority of cardiac patients who become pregnant. In recent years, the incidence of congenital heart disease has increased because of the large number of women with congenital heart lesions that have become treatable, either surgically or medically. Maternal mortality with heart disease ranges from 1 to 17 percent, depending on the severity of disease.[7] Pulmonary edema, due to increased left atrial pressure, accounts for many of the acute emergencies in pregnant cardiac patients. The treatment of this condition is considered after discussing some of the normal cardiovascular changes that occur during pregnancy.

The cardiovascular system adapts during pregnancy to provide for the needs of both the mother and fetus. There is an increase of about 40 to 45 percent in the maternal blood volume. Plasma volume increases early and rapidly, while red cell mass increases more slowly. This produces a "physiologic anemia" during the second trimester which adds stress to the already compromised heart. The cardiac output increases 30 to 40 percent by the end of the first trimester. Only slightly greater values are found in the second and third trimesters. The initial increase in cardiac output is due to an increase in stroke volume. As pregnancy progresses, heart rate increases and stroke volume decreases.

These physiologic changes make it difficult sometimes to determine the normal from the pathologic cardiac exam. The first heart sound becomes louder and the split is exaggerated. S_3 gallops are heard in 84 percent and S_4 gallops in 16 percent of pregnant patients.[8] Systolic murmurs are heard in the majority of patients. Physiologic tricuspid diastolic murmurs are rarely found.

To make the diagnosis of heart disease in pregnancy, one has to differentiate the heart sounds, hyperventilation, dyspnea, and pedal edema normally seen in pregnancy from the pathologic conditions found with cardiac disease. If a patient presents with a diastolic murmur, unequivocal cardiomegaly, Grade III/VI systolic murmur, severe arrythmia, or bilateral basal rales that don't clear with coughing, true cardiac disease is present.

Pulmonary edema may have a sudden onset in the pregnant patient with mitral stenosis. The increased cardiac output elevates the left atrial pressure and the tachycardia shortens the diastolic filling time. Both of these effects will increase further the already expanded pulmonary volume. These factors make the pregnant patient with mitral stenosis prone to pulmonary edema. If any added stress occurs; i.e., atrial fibrillation, exercise, infection, hypotension, hyperthyroidism, labor, or delivery, the stable cardiac patient may decompensate rapidly. These patients have to be monitored carefully during the entire pregnancy. They should be followed every 1 to 2 weeks with special attention paid to the subtle, early signs of pulmonary edema: i.e., a decreased vital capacity or increased pulse rate. Treatment with increasing bed rest in the left lateral position, salt restriction, diuretics, and prophylactic digitalization should be considered. If, despite these measures, the patient still develops pulmonary edema, prompt and effective treatment is needed to preserve fetal as well as maternal well-being.

Effective treatment consists of reducing the cardiac work load, increasing the myocardial contractile force, and reducing congestion. Cardiac work is decreased by decreasing physical activity or eliminating any disease states that increase cardiac work; i.e., infection, or hyperthyroidism. During pregnancy, this may necessitate extended periods of bed rest and possibly hospitalization from the second trimester until term. Effective myocardial contractility must be improved by correcting any arrythmias that result in decreased ventricular filling or pumping. Supraventricular tachycardias are best treated with digitalization. Rapid digitalization can be accomplished by using digoxin, 1.0 to 1.5 mg orally or 0.75 to 1.0 mg IV over 12 to 24 hours. Besides correcting the rapid ventricular response, this therapy will increase myocardial contractility. If, after this therapy, there is no response, propranalol and cardioversion should be considered.

To reduce congestive symptoms, the patient should be treated with rapid acting diuretics. Furosemide, 20 to 80 mg IV, is usually effective in inhibiting reabsorption of chloride in the ascending limb of the loop of Henle. This causes a diuresis within 5 minutes after IV administration. Serum electrolytes, especially $K+$ and $Na+$, should be evaluated frequently when this therapy is instituted. If digitalis and diuretic therapy are being given together, $K+$ supplementation may be needed to avoid digitalis toxicity.

Monitoring of the patient during the episode of pulmonary edema should be accomplished by using a CVP or Swan-Ganz catheter. The latter is usually not necessary because this population of patients does not have intrinsic myocardial disease. Because of this, the CVP is usually an adequate measure of cardiac function.

Fetal well-being is usually not in jeopardy with pulmonary edema unless severe hypoxia or hypotension occurs. Every effort should be made to maintain a pO_2 over 60 mm Hg. Hypotension can be treated by increasing myocardial contractility and correcting arrythmias with rapid ventricular responses. Fetal monitoring should be done during treatment, but efforts to correct fetal distress by rapid surgical delivery when the mother is not stabilized will only jeopardize the mother more. The increased cardiac output and load that occurs in the immediate postpartum period will cause an added stress that may be fatal. Once the maternal situation has improved, with better oxygenation and uterine perfusion, fetal distress may abate and the need for immediate delivery be eliminated.

Once the patient has been stabilized, continued treatment with bed rest, salt restriction, digitalis, and diuretics is indicated. The need for corrective cardiac surgery should then be evaluated. It is usually best to treat the patient with intensive medical therapy first. Only when this fails should cardiac surgery be considered during the pregnancy. Closed mitral valvulotomy is preferred over open heart surgery because the latter carries with it greater maternal as well as fetal mortality rates.[9] If the patient is maintained on medical therapy, continued hospitalization with a planned, well controlled vaginal delivery will result in the best outcome for both the mother and the fetus.

ASTHMA

Asthma during pregnancy has no predictable course. It can worsen, improve, or remain stable. Some patients characteristically improve during the first trimester, but then worsen during the second and third trimesters. Maternal, fetal, or neonatal mortalities related to asthma are rare.[10] This should occur only in patients severely affected and usually only because of inadequate aggressive therapy. If maternal oxygenation can be maintained, fetal hypoxemia will be avoided. This will assure the well-being of the fetus.

Patients who present to the emergency room with symptoms of asthma must be evaluated for other possible diagnoses; i.e., foreign bodies, mucus plugs, pulmonary embolism, or "cardiac asthma." The severity of the attack should be determined by taking a detailed history of the attack. The precipitating event, time of onset, and previous therapy should be documented. A physical examination which documents the presence of wheezing and pulsus paradoxus should be done. Arterial blood gases should be obtained if the patient doesn't respond to therapy quickly. If the pCO_2 is 35 mm Hg and the pH less than 7.40 in the face of hyperventilation, respiratory failure may be imminent. Measurement of the forced expiratory volume in 1 second (FEV_1) by spirometry is helpful in determining the severity and clinical course of an attack. FEV_1 is not changed during pregnancy as compared to the non-pregnant state.[11] FEV_1 is usually less than 1500 cc prior to treatment of the asthmatic attack. If there is any evidence of superimposed infection, a chest x-ray should be obtained. The abdomen can be shielded so that there is no adverse effect on the fetus.

Therapy should be initiated as soon as the diagnosis is confirmed. Successful treatment will produce a decrease in dyspnea and respiratory rate and an increase in FEV_1. The mainstays of therapy are hydration, oxygenation, bronchodilators, and postural drainage. Patients with mild attacks should be treated with aqueous epinephrine, 0.3 to 0.5 ml of 1:1000 dilution subcutaneously every 20 to 30 minutes. If the patient does not respond after 3 doses, IV hydration and bronchodilators should be initiated. The use of epinephrine during pregnancy has been questioned because of its uterine blood vessel constricting effect, but as no evidence of fetal jeopardy has been documented, its use as a first line form of therapy can be continued.

When a patient does not respond to subcutaneous epinephrine, an IV of D5½NS at 200 cc/hr should be started. If the pO_2 is 60 mm Hg or less, O_2 therapy via a moisturized rebreathing system should be initiated. IV aminophylline is the next drug to be used. By inhibiting cAMP, relaxation of bronchial smooth muscles occurs. If the patient has not been taking any theophylline preparations, a loading dose of 5 to 6 mg/Kg is given over 20 to 30 minutes. This is followed by a maintenance dose of 0.4 to 0.9 mg/Kg/hr. The safest way to administer this is by controlled infusion pump. This eliminates the possibility of side effects because of inadvertent high doses.

Inhalation therapy with isoproterenol (0.5 ml of a 1:200 dilution plus 1.5 cc of normal saline) or Bronkosol (0.5 ml) may be given for their nebulizing and bronchodilatation effects. These can usually be given with epinephrine or aminophylline because most pregnant patients with asthma are young and don't have underlying cardiac disease.

When the patient does not respond to these measures, corticosteroids should be used. Hydrocortisone, 250 to 1000 mg as a starting dose, followed by 100 to 300 mg every 4 to 5 hours, can be used in the pregnant patient. There is transfer across the placenta, but this is not a problem. Neonates born after the mother has been treated with high dose steroids for acceleration of fetal lung maturation have not had significant adrenal suppression. The patient will usually improve after steroids within 24 hours. At that time, the dosage can be reduced to 50 to 100 mg IV every 6 hours. After stabilization, prednisone, which crosses the placenta poorly, can be used for maintenance therapy (Table 5.3).

If a patient does not respond to therapy and continues to be hypoxic and retains CO_2, tracheal intubation should be considered. Because maternal hypoxemia will result in fetal hypoxia, maintenance of maternal pO_2 is mandatory. In cases where severe hypoxia has persisted for prolonged periods, intrauterine deaths have resulted.

Once the patient is stabilized, she should be carefully evaluated for any precipitating factors. She should avoid any known allergens. Any underlying respiratory infections should be treated. Chronic therapy with theophylline, beta-2 agonist agents, or steroids can be used during pregnancy. The use of cromolyn sodium in pregnancy has not been fully evaluated, so its use as a prophylactic agent should be reserved for only the most difficult cases.

Table 5-3. Treatment of asthma

1. Epinephrine—0.3–0.5 ml of 1:1000 solution
2. IV therapy—D5½NS at 200 cc/hr
3. Aminophylline—5–6 mg/Kg over 20–30 min, then 0.4–0.9 mg/Kg/hr
4. Inhalation therapy—Isoproterenol or Bronkosol
5. Hydrocortisone—250–1000 mg, then 100–300 mg q 4–5 hr
6. Prednisone—20–60 mg qd. Taper as directed.

PULMONARY EMBOLISM

The risk of thromboembolism is increased 5 to 6 times in the pregnant patient.[12] This increased risk occurs mostly in the postpartum period, but a pulmonary embolus (PE) may occur any time during the pregnancy. The increased risk of pulmonary embolism during pregnancy occurs because of the increase in (1) clotting factors (Vitamin K-dependent factors), (2) venous distensibility, and (3) uterine size, causing decreased venous flow below the vena cava.

The normal pregnant patient experiences dyspnea, tachypnea, and tachycardia. Because these are the cardinal signs of pulmonary embolism, the diagnosis during pregnancy may be difficult. Leg pain, hemoptysis, pleuritic pain, and cough may occur with a pulmonary embolism. Physical diagnosis should be done to look for signs of deep leg vein thrombosis (cords, Homan's sign, erythema, or edema) and right ventricular overload (neck vein distension and fixed splitting of P_2). If the history and/or physical findings are suggestive of pulmonary embolism, ECG and arterial blood gases should be obtained. The ECG findings of right heart strain P-pulmonale, or S_1Q_3 pattern are suggestive. PaO_2 of less than 75 mm Hg is abnormal and is usually confirmatory of the diagnosis. When the diagnosis is still in doubt after these values are obtained, it is usually best to treat the patient with heparin acutely until a lung scan can be obtained. Iodinated radiodiagnostic agents should not be used during pregnancy. These are concentrated 20 to 50 times more in the fetal thyroid (after 12 weeks of gestation) than in the maternal thyroid. Therefore, even small doses may affect fetal thyroid development. Technetium-albumin combinations should be used and give excellent scans. If the scan is equivocal, or fails to confirm a very strong suspicion of embolism, pulmonary angiography, with shielding of the abdomen, can be done.

Once the diagnosis is confirmed or ruled out, the treatment is similar to that in the non-pregnant patient, except Coumadin should not be used during pregnancy. Heparin therapy should be initiated by giving a bolus dose of 5000 to 10,000 units IV. This is followed by keeping the patient on a continuous infusion of 1000 to 1500 units/hr. The rate is adjusted to keep the partial thromboplastin time 2 to 2½ times baseline values. IV heparin should be continued for 7 days. At that time, subcutaneous heparin, 5000 units every 6 to 12 hours, is initiated. This should be continued until delivery. During the early postpartum period, if the patient had a PE during the pregnancy, full IV heparin therapy should be reinstituted. Low dose subcutaneous heparin therapy then can be continued for at least 4 to 6 weeks postpartum.

OTHER MEDICAL EMERGENCIES

Hypertensive emergencies, acute abdominal problems, and bleeding during pregnancy are covered in other chapters. Acute drug overdosage, cardiac arrythmias, thyroid storm, sickle crisis, GI bleeding, and other problems may occur during pregnancy and present to the emergency room physician for initial treatment. After considering the physiologic changes of pregnancy discussed in this and other chapters, treatment can be initiated. Most cases should be treated as if the patient were not pregnant. If necessary diagnostic procedures or effective therapies are withheld, a worsening of the maternal condition, with consequent deterioration of the fetal condition, may result. This is to be avoided at all costs. Once the medical emergency has been successfully diagnosed and treated, the fetal condition will usually be improved.

CONCLUSION

Most medical emergencies that occur during pregnancy can be treated successfully and effectively without longterm morbidity to either the mother or fetus. I have discussed several specific emergencies that are common and have special significance because of physiologic changes that occur during pregnancy. In all cases, maternal well-being and stabilization should be accomplished before any attempt to deliver the fetus is made. This same principle should be applied to all acute emergencies during pregnancy. When maternal survival is in doubt though, despite the best medical therapy, it sometimes becomes necessary to do a cesarean section on a dying or dead mother. Emergency room physicians may have to do, or initiate, this procedure prior to the arrival of a trained surgeon. This can be done with any scalpel. Skin, subcutaneous tissue, and fascia are incised. The peritoneal cavity is then opened. The uterus is incised and the fetus and placenta removed. If the patient is still alive, the uterus, peritoneum and fascia should be closed. The subcutaneous tissue and skin can be left open to heal by secondary intent. This situation arises rarely, but knowledge of this procedure may allow the emergency room physician to be prepared for all obstetrical medical emergencies.

REFERENCES

1. Felig P, Lynch V: Starvation in human pregnancy: hypoglycemia, hypoinsulinemia, and hyperketonemia. Science 170:990, 1970.
2. Page MA, Williamson DH: Enzymes of ketone-body utilization in human brain. Lancet 2:66, 1971.
3. Churchill JA, Berendes HW, Nemare J: Neuropsychological deficits in children of diabetic mothers. Am J Obstet Gynecol 105:257, 1969.
4. Felig P: Diabetes mellitis. p. 185. In Burrows GH, Ferris TF, Eds: Medical Complications During Pregnancy. W.B. Saunders, Philadelphia, 1975.
5. Fisher JN, Shahshahani MD, Kitabchi AE: Diabetic ketoacidosis: low-dose insulin therapy by various routes. N Engl J Med 297:238, 1977.
6. Ueland K: Cardiovascular diseases complicating pregnancy. Clin Obstet Gynecol 21:429, 1978.
7. Szekely P, Snarth L: Atrial fibrillation and pregnancy. Br Med J 1:1407, 196.
8. Cutforth R, MacDonald CB: Heart murmurs in pregnancy. Am Heart J 71:741, 1966.
9. Zitnik RS, Brandenburg RO, Sheldon R, Wallace RB: Pregnancy and open-heart surgery. Circulation 39 (Suppl):1–257, 1969.
10. Bahna SL, Bjerkedal T: The course and outcome of pregnancy in women with bronchial asthma. Acta Allergae 27:397, 1972.
11. Cameron SJ, Bain HH, Grant IWB: Ventilatory function in pregnancy. Scott Med J 15:243, 1970.
12. Seigel DG: Pregnancy, the puerperium and the steroid contraceptive. In Foster C.S., et al, Eds: The Epidemiology of Venous Thrombosis. Mulbank Mem Fund Q 50:15, 1972.

6 Lower Abdominal Pain

Steven J. Sondheimer

Lower abdominal pain in the female is generally a symptom present in patients with gynecologic problems or a selected group of gastrointestinal (GI) problems. However, almost all causes of abdominal pain can occasionally present with varying degrees of lower abdominal pain. In perforation of a peptic ulcer in which spontaneous healing occurs, the leakage of irritative material to the lower peritoneal area can cause lower abdominal pain. Retroperitoneal processes, such as a bleeding aortic aneurysm or pyelonephritis, may atypically have lower abdominal pain, and ureteral colic with a stone lodged near the ureterovesical junction can simulate other more common causes of lower abdominal pain.

There are a number of clinical classifications helpful in approaching the diagnosis of lower abdominal pain in the female. Dividing the patients by age somewhat limits the differential approach.

Menarche in the United States now occurs at a mean age of 13, and it is a relatively late event in puberty, occuring after thelarche and the peak height velocity.[1] Prior to menarche, estrogen is at a lower level and the prepubescent reproductive tract is not prone to many of the more common causes of lower abdominal pain, especially pelvic inflammatory disease (PID).

PEDIATRIC AGE GROUP (TABLE 6.1)

In this group, the most common causes of abdominal pain are GI in origin; they include acute appendicitis, Meckel's diverticulitis, intussusception, and mesenteric adenitis. In addition, such medical conditions as sickle cell disease, lead poisoning, and Henoch-Schönlein purpura may present with abdominal pain. Ovarian cysts and tumors are relatively rare in this age group. Benign

Table 6-1. Abdominal pain in pediatric age group.

1. GI—acute appendicitis, Meckal's diverticulitis, intussusception, mesenteric adenitis
2. Medical—sickle cell disease, lead poisoning, Henoch-Schönlein purpura
3. Gyn—ovarian cysts: rupture & torsion, ovarian tumors: rupture & torsion
4. Congenital abnormalities of Müllerian system—
   imperforate hymen, transverse septum, uterine horn abnormality

cystic teratomas (dermoids) and simple cysts of the ovary (follicular) can be associated with torsion of the pedicle. In addition, remnants of the Wolfian duct system can form cysts which are vulnerable to torsion. Anorexia and vomiting, frequent findings in appendicitis, can also occur with torsion of ovarian cysts. The pain pattern and symptom complex in ovarian torsion is variable from colicky pain to constant unilateral lower abdominal pain. These are surgical emergencies and the correct diagnosis is often not made until laparotomy.

After menarche, the differential diagnosis includes all the possibilities found in the older age group. This is an especially important point since it is necessary to take a complete gynecological and sexual history in a 13 or 14 year old in whom puberty has occurred. One special category is congenital disorders of the Müllerian ductal system. An imperforate hymen can cause cyclic discomfort without visible menstruation. Usually the patient complains of pain worsening over a few months with cycle exacerbations. However, there is a great variation in the pain, from almost no discomfort to constant daily severe lower abdominal pain. A bulging intact hymen, of course, is the clue to diagnosis. The treatment is hospitalization and excision under general anesthesia for optimal results. A transverse septum of the vagina or a non-communicating uterine horn can also present with similar symptoms. The diagnosis and treatment of these conditions is more difficult and requires special surgical skills for proper management. Every pediatric female with lower abdominal pain needs a gynecologic examination.

REPRODUCTIVE AGE GROUP (TABLE 6.2)

In this group, the approach to differential diagnosis can be divided into pregnancy-related and non-pregnancy-related causes of lower abdominal pain. Since pregnancy past the first trimester is more easily diagnosed, I will limit this classification to complications of the first trimester.

Pregnancy-related causes of lower abdominal pain include ectopic pregnancy, threatened abortion, incomplete abortion, round ligament distention, torsion or rupture of a corpus luteum cyst or other ovarian tumor, such as a dermoid cyst. In addition, all of the non-pregnancy-related causes of pelvic

Table 6-2. Abdominal pain in the reproductive age group.

1. Pregnancy related—Ectopic, threatened abortion, incomplete abortion, round ligament pain, torsion or rupture of ovarian cysts or tumors
2. Non-pregnancy related—PID, appendicitis, diverticulitis, endometriosis, torsion or rupture of ovarian cysts or tumors, torsion or degeneration of fibroid tumors, pyelonephritis

pain can occur and must be considered, especially appendicitis. Pelvic inflammatory disease is less common in pregnancy but can occur in the first trimester. Illegal abortions caused many infections in the past but are less frequent today because of the availability of safe medical abortions. Degeneration of a fibroid tumor usually occurs later in the pregnancy, as the fibroid outgrows its blood supply.

Though there is much overlap in symptomatology, the causes of lower abdominal pain not related to pregnancy can be grouped separately. A number of the newer diagnostic tools are important in separating the pregnant from the non-pregnant patient. A common cause of pelvic pain is, of course, pelvic inflammatory disease or salpingitis, either gonococcal or non-gonococcal. The symptoms may be similar to appendicitis, diverticulitis, endometriosis, ectopic pregnancy, torsion of an ovarian cyst or pedunculated fibroid, and pyelonephritis, all of which are important in the differential diagnosis.

The user of an intrauterine contraceptive device (IUD) probably deserves special attention because lower abdominal pain is a common complaint. In the first year of their use, 12 percent of IUD's are removed because of bleeding or pain.[2] In addition, there is a 2 to 7 fold increase in the incidence of pelvic inflammatory disease in IUD users.[3,4] Though the overall rate of ectopic pregnancy is less in IUD wearers than in non-contracepting females, the chances of a pregnancy being ectopic in an IUD wearer is greater. A number of cases of unilateral salpingitis with tubo-ovarian abscess or sepsis have been reported in pregnant and non-pregnant IUD wearers.[5,6]

POSTMENOPAUSAL AGE GROUP (TABLE 6.3)

Appendicitis and tubo-ovarian abscess formation can occur in this group, though less frequently than in younger women, and because of this, these disorders are often diagnosed late in their course. Left-sided lower abdominal pain with fever is suggestive of diverticulitis, but other diagnoses include carcinoma of the colon and torsion of an adnexa. Such gastrointestinal disorders as volvulis, mesenteric vascular occlusion, and small bowel obstruction from internal hernia or adhesions can also cause lower abdominal pain.

Table 6-3. Abdominal pain in the postmenopausal age group.

1. Appendicitis
2. Tuboovarian abscess
3. Diverticulitis
4. Carcinoma of the colon
5. Torsion of adnexa
6. GI—volvulus, mesenteric vascular occlusion, small bowel obstruction

Table 6-4. Symptoms of ectopic pregnancy.

1. Abdominal pain
2. Vaginal bleeding
3. Symptoms of pregnancy—amenorrhea, nausea, breast tenderness
4. Orthostatic symptoms—fainting, shock, dizziness

ECTOPIC PREGNANCY (TABLE 6.4)

An ectopic pregnancy is a pregnancy which occurs in a location other than the uterine cavity. Ninety-five percent of these pregnancies occur within the fallopian tube. Ectopic pregnancy is one of the major causes of maternal mortality in the United States today. In 1978, there were 12 direct maternal deaths in Philadelphia; 4 of these deaths were due to ruptured ectopic pregnancies.

A majority of patients who develop a ruptured ectopic pregnancy are seen by a physician and referred out prior to their eventual hospitalization. Our goal should be the identification and treatment of the unruptured tubal pregnancy. This will minimize the risk of bleeding and its complications; in addition, though a bit more controversial, such treatment will allow for preservation of the involved fallopian tube and possibly increase fertility potential. Patients whose first pregnancy is ectopic have a poor subsequent reproductive potential.[7] In one report of 50 such females, 24 percent developed subsequent ectopic pregnancies and only 30 percent produced live births.[8]

Normal uterine implantation occurs approximately 7 days after ovulation. The fertilized egg remains within the fallopian tube for 3 days and within the uterine cavity prior to implantation another 4 days. Implantation occurs at the time the embryo has divided into a blastocyst. With trophoblastic differentiation at approximately 7 days after ovulation, human chorionic gonadotropin (HCG), is first detectable in blood by a sensitive radioimmune assay specific for the beta subunit of this glycoprotein. A tubal pregnancy may occur if the ovum is delayed in its transport through the tube, allowing development of the trophoblastic layer to occur.

The major disaster of ectopic pregnancies, of course, is intra-abdominal bleeding. This is usually due to the erosive action of the trophoblast, with subsequent tubal rupture and bleeding from the tube or mesosalpinx. Occasionally, intraluminal bleeding occurs with bleeding from the fimbriated end; this type of bleeding is usually less brisk. The most catastrophic blood loss occurs with rupture near the uterus, as can occur with an interstitial pregnancy. Unfortunately, these are also often the most difficult ectopic pregnancies to diagnose early.

James L. Breen, at St. Barnabas Hospital in Livingston, New Jersey, describes a large series of ectopic pregnancies.[9] Eighty percent of the patients in that series had a ruptured fallopian tube at operation. Approximately 40 percent of the patients had 1 to 2 units of blood in the abdomen; 8 percent had over 1500 cc of blood intra-abdominally.

Previous tubal infection is a major etiologic factor in ectopic pregnancy. Fully 25 percent of patients have a history of pelvic inflammatory disease, and 50 percent of fallopian tubes removed because of an ectopic pregnancy will show pathologic evidence of prior inflammatory disease. Lars Westrum, in Sweden, followed 415 patients with a laparoscopically diagnosed pelvic inflammatory disease. Three hundred and fifty of these women subsequently attempted to conceive; 3.4 percent of them developed ectopic pregnancies. Of the pregnancies which occurred in this group, 1 in 24 was ectopic.[10]

Pelvic tuberculosis [11] is rare in the United States. Very few pregnancies occur after pelvic TB and those that occur are usually ectopic in location.

Thirty percent of infertility is due to tubal disease; adhesions, old inflammatory disease, or endometriosis. These patients are at an increased risk of ectopic pregnancy. Many patients with ectopic pregnancies will have a longstanding history of infertility. In addition, those who have had tubal surgery to restore fertility have an increased risk of ectopic pregnancy.

The incidence of repeat ectopic pregnancy ranges from 10 to 25 percent.

Ectopic pregnancies can occur following tubal sterilization surgery. In a recent review of 100 consecutive ectopic pregnancy patients, 7 of them had a previous tubal ligation, 3 by tubal fulguration.[12,13]

Previous appendicitis is probably responsible for the higher incidence of right-sided ectopic pregnancies.

It has been suggested that the IUD is responsible for the recent increased incidence of ectopic pregnancies. This is probably not true. IUD wearers have a lower incidence of ectopic pregnancies than do non-contracepting females; however, the IUD protects better against intrauterine pregnancies than ectopic pregnancies. Short-term users have a lower incidence of ectopic pregnancy than long-term users of the IUD. There is no difference in risks between copper devices and plastic devices. Approximately 1 out of 25 pregnancies which occur with the IUD in place will be ectopic.[14]

The common problem in the IUD user of vaginal bleeding and abdominal pain takes on additional concern because of the always present risk of ectopic pregnancy. The sensitive serum pregnancy test should be ordered often in the IUD wearer with abdominal complaints.

The progesterone-only birth control pill, which is used in women who are at risk from the estrogen in the combination pill, protects less well against tubal pregnancies than intrauterine pregnancies; therefore, as with the IUD, there is less ectopic pregnancy than in non-contraceptors but a higher ratio of ectopic to intrauterine pregnancies than normal.

After an elective first trimester abortion, an occasional patient will return to the emergency room with abdominal pain or bleeding. Ectopic pregnancy should be considered in the differential diagnosis and it is important to check the original pathology report to confirm that products of contraception, i.e. trophoblastic material, were seen at the time of the abortion.

In summary, any woman in the reproductive age group who is sexually active and not using the combination birth control pill is at risk for an ectopic pregnancy.

Only about 15 percent of patients present to the emergency room with a classic history and examination for an ectopic pregnancy. What is that history? A 20 year old sexually active female, who is not using the combination birth control pill, complains of initial amenorrhea followed 1 to 2 weeks later with abnormal vaginal "spotting" or bleeding, usually scantier than normal. She then notes the sudden onset of abdominal pain or the acute exacerbation of a previously present sharp or dull pain, unilaterally, in the lower abdominal area.

She then experiences shoulder pain (diaphragmatic irritation from intra-abdominal blood). She also gives a history of orthostatic dizziness and possibly a syncopal episode. On physical exam, this patient may have a temperature of about 99°F and will have signs of shock; that is, cold, clammy skin with a thready pulse and low blood pressure. There is lower abdominal tenderness. Pelvic examination shows unilateral tenderness and guarding in the adnexal area, with pain on motion of the cervix. The cervix may be soft and cyanotic, suggestive of pregnancy. The cul-de-sac is bulging with a doughy consistency.

There is no question in a patient who presents with this type of history and examination that she has an ectopic pregnancy and is in shock secondary to intra-abdominal bleeding; however, most patients do not present with such a classic history.

Abdominal and pelvic pain is the most consistent finding in women with ectopic pregnancy. All of the patients in Breen's series complained of some degree of abdominal pain. However, in very early ectopic pregnancies, this may be found less frequently. On questioning, however, most patients will remember mild, crampy to sharp lower abdominal pain prior to an acute exacerbation. The pain is described as sharp and colicky, often unilateral but not always. Occasionally, patients will complain of a constant urge to defecate, especially if the tubal mass is pushing against the rectum. The patient's pain may present atypically. In Breen's series, 10 percent of patients complained of shoulder pain, 5 percent of back pain, 10 percent of pain in the entire abdomen, and 20 percent of pain in the opposite quadrant from the side of the eventual ectopic pregnancy. Vaginal bleeding is an even more variable symptom. In Breen's series, 84 percent of patients did experience amenorrhea and 80 percent had some degree of irregular vaginal bleeding. Most of these patients described the abnormal bleedings as scant, though a large number chose moderate, and a little less than 10 percent described the bleeding as profuse. Of interest in this group with profuse vaginal bleeding, 9 out of 43 patients had an interstitial pregnancy.

Some women will have noted such early symptoms of pregnancy as nausea and breast tenderness. Often these symptoms disappear before the tube ruptures.

The patient in shock is no diagnostic problem, but an occasional patient will have fainted at home during an episode of pain or have noted some marked orthostatic dizziness. All patients except those in shock should be examined in the supine and then in the standing or sitting position. A drop in blood pressure with an increase in pulse suggests hypovolemia. Maternal mortalities have occurred in patients admitted to the intensive care unit unconscious secondary to a fall in the bathroom at home, and then discovered to have an undiagnosed ruptured ectopic pregnancy.

On physical exam, the patient is usually afebrile or has a temperature between 99 and 100°F. This low grade temperature may be due to abdominal bleeding. Seldom does a temperature go above 101°F as is found in pelvic inflammatory disease, though occasionally a higher temperature is encountered.[9]

Abdominal and pelvic tenderness are probably the most consistent physical findings. The cervix may be soft and cyanotic and the uterus slightly enlarged. Unilateral adnexal tenderness is common but occasionally the tenderness is bilateral and there is pain on motion of the cervix. A mass may or may not be present. Usually there is just a suggestion of a fullness, and even when a mass is palpated, it is often the corpus luteum that is being felt. The ectopic is often too soft and tender to allow clear delineation. A pelvic hematocele may be present from blood in the cul-de-sac.

A normal white blood cell count or occasionally a mild leukocytosis is present. The hemoglobin level and hematocrit usually correlate well with the degree of hematoperitoneum. Changes in hemoglobin from a previous known value may be helpful.[9]

Forty percent of patients with ectopic pregnancies will have a negative urine pregnancy test by the 2 minute latex agglutination slide test, which has a sensitivity for HCG of 1500 mIU/ml. However, the serum radioreceptor assay for HCG is sensitive for HCG to 200 mIU/ml, and in one series, 66 of 70 patients with proven ectopic pregnancies had a positive test (in contrast, only 82 percent of patients had a positive culdocentesis and 69 percent a positive urine pregnancy test).[15] In that series, of the four patients with negative tests, two were in shock and had positive culdocentesis, one had an ectopic pregnancy noted at elective cuff salpingostomy, and one other had a chronic ectopic pregnancy. Probably all patients with an ectopic pregnancy will have evidence of HCG in the blood detectable by a RIA-HCG serum assay. However, a positive pregnancy test does not differentiate an intrauterine pregnancy (IUP) from an ectopic pregnancy, nor does quantitative testing of serum HCG or progesterone adequately differentiate an ectopic pregnancy from a threatened abortion.

Pelvic gray-scale ultrasound may be helpful if it shows a clearcut gestational sac within the uterine cavity. The gestational sac usually becomes visible on gray-scale ultrasound 5 weeks from the last normal menstrual period (LNMP). If the gestational sac is seen within the uterine cavity, then an ectopic pregnancy is probably not present. However, there is a 1 in 30,000 risk of a simultaneous ectopic and intrauterine pregnancy. Occasionally mild intrauterine bleeding with a decidual endometrial reaction can produce a picture resembling a gestational sac on ultrasound.[16] In addition, a pregnancy within the interstitial portion of the tube may be interpreted as an intrauterine pregnancy.

Kelly et al reported on the use of gray-scale ultrasound in diagnosis of ectopic pregnancy.[17] Fifty-nine ectopic pregnancies were diagnosed without ultrasound. Of 260 patients referred for ultrasound, 94 out of 260 had a definite intrauterine pregnancy identified, and there was no false positive here. Five of 99 intrauterine pregnancies could not be identified on ultrasound, probably because the pregnancy was too early. Seventeen of 25 ectopic pregnancies were correctly identified. However, 10 patients with ectopic pregnancies were not identified, though no gestational sac was seen either. In conclusion, pelvic ultrasound is valuable if an intrauterine pregnancy is clearly identified.

Culdocentesis allows direct sampling of the peritoneal cavity for evidence of a hematoperitoneum. It is usually performed with a patient in the dorsal lithotomy position. If the patient is clinically stable, it helps to put the head of the bed up in order to fill the cul-de-sac. A #18 gauge spinal needle is inserted into the posterior fornix between the uterosacral ligaments at the site of maximum distention. The vagina can be infiltrated with 1 percent lidocaine. However, adequate anesthesia of the peritoneum is not often accomplished, and usually it is just as well to do the procedure without local anesthesia. The needle is attached to a 10cc syringe and directed horizontally to avoid perforation of the rectum or sigmoid. The finding of non-clotting blood means that bleeding into the peritoneal cavity has occurred. If pus is obtained, it can be sent for gram stain, aerobic and anaerobic cultures. Clotting blood usually implies that a vessel of the uterus or vagina has been entered. However, brisk bleeding from a ruptured ectopic can occasionally cause clotted blood to be obtained. A negative tap means that peritoneal fluid is obtained without blood. The absence of aspirated fluid is a non-diagnostic tap and cannot be interpreted as a negative tap. Culdocentesis should not be attempted if a cul-de-sac mass is palpated or if the uterus is severely retroflexed and cannot be mobilized anteriorly.

What is the place for culdocentesis? Should every patient with any suspicion of an ectopic pregnancy undergo culdocentesis? Most importantly, will the results of the culdocentesis change the management of the patient? Breen's policy at St. Barnabas Hospital was for all patients with a suspicion of ectopic pregnancy to undergo culdocentesis. Out of 654 patients with an ectopic pregnancy, 591 had a confirmatory culdocentesis, which allowed for efficient management of the patients. However, in his series, 80 percent of the patients had a ruptured ectopic pregnancy. In patients with signs and symptoms of an ectopic pregnancy and obvious shock or with significant orthostatic changes, it is not necessary to do a culdocentesis in the emergency room. These patients will need laparotomy, so they should be stabilized and efficiently transported to the operating room. In the operating room, the decision can be made on whether to proceed with a culdocentesis. The patient in whom an ectopic pregnancy is suspected, who is completely stable, with minimal pain and no anemia or no orthostatic changes, can be managed by close observation, sensitive serum pregnancy test, and pelvic ultrasound and laparoscopy as indicated; culdocentesis probably will not be helpful in this type of patient.

Patients with equivocal signs of orthostasis, with anemia in whom other diagnostic procedures are not readily available, and in whom the diagnosis of pelvic inflammatory disease versus ectopic pregnancy is considered, may benefit from culdocentesis. However, a non-diagnostic culdocentesis is not helpful. A positive culdocentesis requires at least a laparoscopy, but a negative culdocentesis probably allows for close observation of the patient while awaiting the availability of further diagnostic procedures.

Laparoscopy is one of the major advances in gynecology in the last decade. It affords relatively safe visualization of the pelvis. Diagnostic laparoscopy is best performed under general anesthesia, with endotracheal intubation.

Adequate visualization of the entire pelvis requires a two puncture technique, with the laparoscope inserted through the umbilicus and a second wand introduced in the lower abdominal area.

An absolute contraindication to laparoscopy is a distended abdomen secondary to bowel obstruction or ileus. Relative contraindications include previous surgery, massive obesity, hiatal hernia, and inflammatory bowel disease. In the moribund patient with obvious intra-abdominal bleeding, valuable time is wasted in visualization of a hemoperitoneum.

Laparoscopy is the best diagnostic procedure short of exploratory laparotomy. However, occasionally laparoscopy will not allow adequate visualization of the fallopian tube, and laparotomy will be necessary. Also, an early ectopic pregnancy or an interstitial pregnancy can be missed at laparoscopy. In addition, at laparoscopy, if the tube appears edematous from pelvic inflammatory disease, it may be necessary to do a laparotomy to evaluate the possibility of an ectopic tubal pregnancy. However, laparoscopy is still the single most important asset in early diagnosis of the ectopic pregnancy.

Laparoscopy is especially helpful in patients with pelvic pain, either acute or chronic, in whom the differential diagnosis includes endometriosis or pelvic adhesions. Although a diagnostic and therapeutic D&C is often performed prior to a laparoscopy, the only time a D&C is useful is if the differential diagnosis includes an incomplete abortion. In that case, if trophoblastic material is found, the likelihood of a simultaneous ectopic is 1 in 30,000. If the patient desires an abortion, a D&C can be done first as a diagnostic as well as therapeutic procedure. The endometrium in cases of surgically proven ectopic pregnancies may show secretory, proliferative, menstrual, or a decidual pattern. The Arias-Stella reaction is an endometrial picture of hypersecretory glands with vaculated cytoplasm and atypical nuclei. This endometrial histology, in different series, is noted in 5 to 75 percent of patients with an ectopic pregnancy.[18] It is a difficult pathologic diagnosis to make and it can also be seen with a complete abortion. If a patient has had an elective abortion and the pathology does not demonstrate chorionic villi or fetal parts, then that patient should be seen immediately and evaluated for possible ectopic pregnancy.

Prompt diagnosis of an ectopic pregnancy requires always considering this diagnosis in any woman of childbearing age with abdominal pain. In patients with a suspected ectopic pregnancy, we can divide the differential diagnosis into two categories: complications of an early pregnancy with similar symptoms, and conditions with similar symptoms not associated with pregnancy.

COMPLICATIONS OF EARLY PREGNANCY WITH SIMILAR SYMPTOMS

Threatened abortion or an incomplete abortion can present with pain and vaginal bleeding quite similar to an ectopic pregnancy. If the internal cervical os is open, then a D&C is necessary. Gray-scale ultrasound should be able to localize a gestational sac within the uterus by 5 weeks from the LNMP. Real-time ultrasound will demonstrate fetal movement by 9 weeks from the LNMP and is a reliable indicator of a viable pregnancy.[19] Since pain from round ligament distention occurs later in the first trimester, ultrasound is usually helpful. Bleeding or torsion from a corpus luteum or other ovarian cyst is an operative emergency so the diagnosis is made at surgery.

If a sensitive serum pregnancy test does not demonstrate HCG, it is unlikely that either an IUP or an ectopic pregnancy exists. In the emergency room setting, differentiating between an ectopic pregnancy and pelvic inflammatory disease is usually the most difficult problem and the source of the greatest potential disaster. Many of the patients with ectopic pregnancies have a history of pelvic inflammatory disease and, therefore, when they appear with pelvic pain, they can be too easily dismissed as recurrent pelvic inflammatory disease. All patients with a diagnosis of afebrile pelvic inflammatory disease require close observation, a sensitive serum pregnancy test, and probably also culdocentesis. Anovulatory bleeding frequently can present with a bleeding pattern suggestive of an ectopic pregnancy. Patients with polycystic ovarian disease often have slightly tender and enlarged ovaries. However, in these patients, a sensitive pregnancy test will be quite helpful. Corpus luteal cysts, particularly hemorrhagic ones, may require laparotomy because of pain and bleeding. A follicular cyst, especially at mid-cycle, may be suggestive of an ectopic pregnancy. Some patients will have vaginal spotting at the time of ovulation. In addition, they may have some mild peritoneal signs from the irritative effect of the follicular fluid in the peritoneum. Other diagnostic considerations include appendicitis and torsion of an ovarian cyst, both surgical emergencies themselves, as well as non-surgical emergencies such as ovarian tumor, fibroids, endometriosis, and pelvic adhesions.

EMERGENCY ROOM MANAGEMENT OF THE RUPTURED ECTOPIC PREGNANCY [20]

The acute management of the patient in shock with significant blood loss from a ruptured ectopic pregnancy first depends on making the diagnosis. A normal, healthy woman in an emergency room situation will have a slight increase in blood pressure when she changes from the supine to the upright position. If there is some pain associated with this movement, there will also be an increase in the pulse. Though the diastolic blood pressure better approximates the mean blood pressure, it is often easier to hear clear-cut changes in the sounds of the systolic blood pressure. A drop of 10 to 20 mm of mercury in blood pressure and a pulse increase of 10 to 20 beats per minute is significant. Again, our young, healthy female, after donating 1 unit of blood, will have minimal or no orthostatic blood pressure changes. Orthostatic blood pressure changes in most young, healthy females probably represent a greater than 10 percent intravascular fluid loss (low blood pressure in the supine position; i.e., shock, usually means, in the young, healthy female, greater than a 20 percent blood loss).

A large bore IV should be started, at least a 16 gauge needle, and occasionally 2 peripheral IV's are needed. If a peripheral IV cannot be started, a subclavian catheter should be inserted. A hemoglobin and hematocrit should be obtained and blood sent for crossmatch. A Foley catheter is inserted and urine output monitored. The most important aspect of initial care, after making the diagnosis, is expansion of intravascular fluid volume to improve the blood pressure.

There is debate concerning the proper fluid to increase vascular volume. At least initially, normal saline is as good as a balanced salt solution such as Normosol or Ringer's Lactate. Saline should be given at such a rate as to restore the blood pressure to a minimally normal level, which may be best determined by the elimination of orthostasis and by the maintenance of an adequate urine output (30–50 cc/hour). Fluid overload, which is usually more of an intraoperative or postoperative problem, can be avoided if care is taken to monitor blood pressure and urine output and to listen to the lungs for rales. If the patient begins to go into congestive heart failure, the blood pressure may begin to fall and the pulse rate increase, but one can avoid being fooled into forcing more fluids by noting an adequate urine output and the onset of rales in the chest. In addition, prior to this point, if a CVP catheter is in place, a rise in central venous pressure will be noted.

Though blood needs to be crossmatched as quickly as possible, remember that in the young, healthy woman, it is blood pressure which initially is the principal concern rather than the hemoglobin loss. Oxygenation can be maintained at a 50 percent hemoglobin loss by increasing cardiac output 2 times. Even a 75 percent loss of hemoglobin requires only a four-fold increase in cardiac output to maintain adequate tissue oxygenation. This is similar to the change in the cardiac output which occurs while playing doubles in tennis.

PELVIC INFLAMMATORY DISEASE

In the United States, there are approximately 1 million new cases of gonorrhea each year in females. Approximately 400,000 cases of salpingitis occur yearly, half secondary to gonorrhea. Unlike the relative success in control of syphilis, the reservoir of asymptomatic male and female carriers of gonorrhea has made eradication very difficult. It is important to remember that all male contacts of a gonococcal (GC) positive female should be treated, whether or not they have symptoms. In addition, contacts of non-gonococcal salpingitis patients should be tested for gonorrhea.[21,22]

If not treated, 15 to 30 percent of women with gonorrhea of the cervix will develop salpingitis. In addition, any procedure which promotes bacterial contamination of the uterine cavity can be an etiologic factor in PID. A recent D&C, D&E, hysterosalpingogram or IUD insertion can be responsible for GC or non-GC salpingitis.[23]

Though classically pelvic inflammatory disease is divided into two types, gonococcal and non-gonococcal, this distinction is less helpful in approaching the emergency room patient. If the diagnosis of PID is made, then treatment should be adequate to cover gonococcus as well as the mixed flora often found in non-gonococcal infections.

An initial gonococcal salpingitis may injure the endosalpinx, predisposing the patient either at this time or in the future to super-infection by anaerobic or aerobic bowel flora. *Chlamydia trachomatis* may also play a significant role in PID.[24] The end stage of pelvic inflammation is pelvic scarring and tubal damage responsible for infertility and chronic lower abdominal pain and tenderness, often without an acute inflammatory process. The diagnostic danger is that salpingitis predisposes to ectopic pregnancy, and these patients with an ectopic pregnancy are often dismissed without proper evaluation because of their past history. In addition, too often because of social, economic, and racial generalizations, patients with endometriosis receive repeated antibiotic courses for misdiagnosed PID.

The classic history for acute salpingitis is bilateral lower abdominal pain beginning just after the onset of the menses, with fever and vaginal discharge. On physical exam, the temperature is over 100°F, there is lower abdominal tenderness and guarding, and on pelvic exam, there is bilateral tenderness of the adnexae with exquisite tenderness on motion of the cervix. The laboratory findings include leukocytosis and elevated erythrocyte sedimentation rate (ESR). Only 20 percent of patients with well-documented PID will present with this history. These patients most often have gonorrheal salpingitis, respond quickly to therapy, and have a relatively good prognosis.

In an outstanding and much needed study from Sweden, Jacobson and Westrum reported on the accuracy of clinical criteria alone in the diagnosis of acute pelvic inflammatory disease.[25] In 814 patients in whom acute PID was suspected, diagnostic laparoscopy was performed. Their criteria for the visual diagnosis of acute salpingitis was hyperemia of the tubal surface, edema of the tubal wall, and a sticky exudate on the tubal surface and from the fimbriated end if patent. In 65 percent of the patients, the diagnosis was confirmed. In 98 cases, 12 percent, other pathology was noted, and in 184 cases, 23 percent, no pathology was noted. A number of the patients with no visual pathology had GC of the endocervix, and it is likely that many of these patients had early salpingitis, parametritis, or endometritis. This, however, still leaves 12 percent who clearly had another pathologic diagnosis.

In the group with laparoscopically confirmed salpingitis, the following frequency of symptoms was reported: lower abdominal pain—94 percent, increased vaginal discharge—55 percent, temperature greater than 38°C or chills—41 percent, irregular vaginal bleeding—36 percent, urinary symptoms—19 percent, vomiting—10 percent, and proctitis symptoms—7 percent. Eshenbach and Holmes observed 31 percent of patients with pelvic infection to have perihepatitis diagnosed by right upper quadrant tenderness. Only a few patients had the characteristic pleuritic upper abdominal pain. Patients with gonococcal salpingitis were more likely than those with non-gonococcal salpingitis to have vaginal discharge and fever and to have the onset of symptoms related to the menses. As Eschenbach and Holmes have noted, there is a spectrum of clinical symptoms in salpingitis, from early salpingitis with no fever and mild abdominal tenderness to the full blown picture with severe lower abdominal pain and fever.[23] Falk noted unilateral salpingitis in 8 percent of his laparoscoped patients with PID. Unilateral tubo-ovarian abscess, and unilateral salpingitis has also been seen occasionally in patients with IUD associated infection.[26]

PID can occur during the first trimester of pregnancy. In the past, septic illegal abortions were the cause of many of these cases. It is probably still wise to obtain a flat plate and erect x-ray film of the abdomen to look for air under the diaphragm, or a foreign object in the uterus or abdomen from a "back alley" abortion.

Leukocytosis is present in only about one-half of the cases of acute PID, and the ESR is elevated in about 75 percent.[23] The WBC and ESR does correlate with severity of the infection and the response to treatment. Though the ESR may stay elevated for a period after apparently successful treatment, this may represent continued inflammation.

Gram stain of the endocervix is not helpful in most cases. If clearcut gram negative diplocci are seen within neutrophils by an experienced pathologist, the diagnosis can be made. In most EW settings, this technique has a low yield. A culture of GC from the endocervix requires specialized transport media or direct plating onto Thayer-Martins media and prompt placement in a candle jar. Except for a GC culture, there is no need for any routine bacterial culture of the vagina or endocervix. Except for GC, there is no relationship between organisms cultured from within the peritoneal cavity in PID patients and those cultured from the endocervix.[27]

Culdocentesis has been advocated for better specific microbiologic identification of implicated organisms. If pus is obtained, it should be gram stained and cultured aerobically and anaerobically. A culdocentesis should not be performed if a mass is present in the cul-de-sac. The most commonly isolated organisms besides *N. gonorrhoeae* are the aerobes *E. coli,* enterococcus, and Group B streptococcus; and the anaerobes peptostreptococcus and *Bacteroides fragilis.*[23,27] Because this information affects one's therapeutic approach infrequently, culdocentesis is more helpful as a check for a hematoperitoneum than as a check for infection.

Both Falk and Westrum and Jacobson have demonstrated that laparoscopy can be safely performed in acute PID.[25,26] As has been noted, 12 percent of patients had other pathology diagnosed at laparoscopy. Of these 98 patients with other diagnosis, the following pathology was found: 24 cases of acute appendicitis, 16 cases of pelvic endometriosis, 12 cases of hemorrhagic corpus luteum, 11 ectopic pregnancies, 7 ovarian tumors, 6 cases of pelvic adhesions, 6 cases of mesenteric lymphadenitis, and 16 other diagnoses. This group did not differ from the group with acute salpingitis in the number or distribution of symptoms or signs. Of interest is a group of 51 patients who had laparoscopic examinations with other preoperative diagnosis who were noted to have acute PID. In 1/3 of these patients, no abdominal pain was reported, and 1/2 had no tenderness on bimanual exam. The preoperative diagnoses included ovarian tumor (11), ectopic pregnancy (15), pelvic adhesions (7); another 17 patients at laparotomy for suspected acute appendicitis were noted to have salpingitis. Liberal use of diagnostic laparoscopy should be encouraged. Laparoscopy is contraindicated when abdominal distention secondary to ileus or bowel obstruction is present or suspected.

In the pre-antibiotic era, most cases of acute PID improved without surgery. However, 15 percent of the patients had prolonged or progressive symptoms. Antibiotics have decreased such serious sequela of PID as pelvic abscess, peritonitis, and tubal occlusion. Antibiotics, then, are the mainstay of therapy. However, a number of questions are still to be answered: (1) which antibiotic regimen is best and by what route; (2) which patients, if not all, should be hospitalized; and (3) when is surgery indicated? Considering the frequency of incorrect diagnosis, some people advocate hospitalizing all patients with PID. In addition, it is possible that parenteral antibiotics may decrease the incidence of serious sequela and infertility. However, at least as a minimum, all patients in whom the diagnosis of PID is in doubt or in whom outpatient antibiotic treatment does not give quick resolution of symptoms should be hospitalized. Patients who may not be able easily to return for a second examination within 24 to 48 hours should be hospitalized. In addition, the usual criteria for hospital admissions and parenteral antibiotic therapy for PID are: (1) inability to do an adequate pelvic exam to rule out an abscess; (2) presence or suspicion of a pelvic or abdominal abscess; (3) four quadrant peritoneal signs; that is, possible peritonitis or a surgical emergency; (4) temperature over 101°F; (5) inability to tolerate or follow an outpatient regimen; (6) failure to respond to outpatient regimen; or (7) pregnancy.

Shown (Table 6.5) is the Center for Disease Control (CDC) recommendation for outpatient management of PID. The regimen includes sufficient coverage for endocervical GC as well as continued antibiotic coverage for salpingitis. If an IUD is present, after the initial dose of antibiotic, it should be removed. Though the effect of removing the IUD on the response to acute salpingitis is unknown, it makes good sense that adequate treatment of an infection cannot be achieved in the presence of a foreign body. Tetracycline, 0.5 g orally, 4 times a day for 10 days, should not be used for pregnant patients. Aqueous procaine penicillin G 4.8 m unit IM, ampicillin 3.5 g or amoxycillin 3.0 g, each with probenecid 1.0 g, are the suggested initial therapies. These regimens are followed by ampicillin or amoxycillin 0.5 g orally 4 times a day for 10 days.[28]

Adequate early treatment of an infection decreases late sequelae. Therefore, it makes good clinical sense to begin therapy early in PID even when the diagnosis is in doubt and the patient is being further evaluated. However, often patients who are told they have PID when the diagnosis of lower abdominal

Table 6-5. Outpatient treatment of PID.

1. Aqueous procaine penicillin 4.8 million units IM + Probenicid 1 g PO then Ampicillin 0.5 g PO qid × 10 days
2. Ampicillin 3.5 g or Amoxycillin 3.0 g + Probenecid 1 g PO then Ampicillin 0.5 g PO qid × 10 days
3. Tetracycline—500 mg PO qid × 10 days

pain is in doubt are treated and discharged from the emergency room. These patients actually need extensive evaluation and followup. Culdocentesis, ultrasound, sensitive serum pregnancy tests, and diagnostic laparoscopy should be especially encouraged in this group of patients. The woman who is repeatedly treated in the clinic and EW for "afebrile" PID or chronic salpingitis probably needs a diagnostic laparoscopy. It is not surprising to find endometriosis or even a normal pelvis in this setting.

TORSION OF THE OVARY OR FALLOPIAN TUBE [29]

Most commonly, torsion occurs with an adnexal mass greater than 6 cm in diameter. In one large series of 135 women with torsion, only 4 normal ovaries and 3 normal fallopian tubes underwent torsion. Usually, a benign ovarian tumor such as a dermoid or a simple cyst of the ovary will be found, but approximately 20 percent of the ovarian masses which undergo torsion will be malignant. Either a paraovarian cyst or an hydrosalpinx is responsible for most tubal torsions.

Patients present with a complaint of acute lower abdominal pain; the pain varies in location from the flank to the groin and also radiates occasionally to the thigh on the involved side. The patients describe the pain as a dull ache with acute exacerbations of sharp pain. Nausea and vomiting may be present with the acute exacerbation. Though abnormal bleeding is not usually present, it can rarely occur in these patients. Interestingly, many patients relate a past history of similar pain which lasted hours to days.

Eighty percent of patients had a palpable tender adnexal mass in the series from the Mayo Clinic. There was often abdominal guarding on the involved side with pain on motion of the cervix. Ninety percent of the patients were afebrile and only 30 percent had a white count greater than 10,000. Patients may have blood on culdocentesis, or serosanguinous fluid. Torsion of the adnexa can occur in pregnancy, especially from an enlarged corpus luteum or dermoid cyst.

If torsion is left untreated, necrosis of the involved organs can lead to peritonitis and shock. Torsion of the fallopian tube or ovary can occur at any age, including infancy and even as an antenatal event.[30] In addition, torsion of the remaining adnexa can occur in the post hysterectomy patient.[31]

Diagnostic laparoscopy should be liberally applied to help in early diagnosis. In a well-equipped hospital, the risks of diagnostic laparoscopy are small compared to the benefit of early diagnosis. A strong case can be made that no patient should leave the emergency room with a diagnosis of pelvic inflammatory disease who has unilateral adnexal tenderness and especially who is afebrile. Those patients deserve further evaluation and observation including possible laparoscopy. This should reduce the incidence of missed ectopic pregnancies and adnexal torsion.

Necrosis of a leiomyoma may occur because of torsion of its pedicle. In addition, carneous or hemorrhagic degeneration of a fibroid can occur spontaneously or when these tumors complicate pregnancy. This acute event may be associated with abdominal pain, tenderness, fever, and leukocytosis.

The treatment of the degenerating fibroid in pregnancy is observation with symptomatic analgesia as necessary. Except for the pedunculated myoma, myomectomy is too dangerous a procedure in the pregnant uterus. The frequency of degeneration during pregnancy is secondary to alterations in the blood supply as the myoma grows under estrogen stimulation. Degeneration is more common in the second or third trimester or in the post abortive or postpartum period.

ENDOMETRIOSIS

The pain of endometriosis is usually bilateral lower abdominal in location, with premenstrual or menstrual aggravation. Most patients have a history of dysmenorrhea. Other symptoms can include dyspareunia, pain on defecation, premenstrual spotting, dysuria or hematuria, and infertility. Endometriomas or endometriotic cysts may rupture or leak, causing peritoneal irritation with severe pain and peritoneal signs. Endometriosis cannot be diagnosed by history and physical examination alone. Specific treatment for endometriosis should not usually be undertaken without laparoscopic or histiologic confirmation.

APPENDICITIS [32]

Appendicitis can occur at any age but is most common from the early teens until 30. However, it can be most devastating in the very young or the old since it usually is not suspected early.

Classically, appendicitis presents with periumbilical or generalized abdominal pain which then, over a number of hours, localizes to the right lower quadrant. Abdominal pain is the most frequent finding, followed by anorexia, then nausea and vomiting. Constipation is more common than diarrhea, which, however, can also occur. With variation in position of the appendix, pain and tenderness may be found in the left lower quadrant, the suprapubic area, the cul-de-sac and rectum, or the flank.

In the female, the most common problem in diagnosis is with PID. Anorexia and GI complaints are more common in appendicitis. Fever may be higher in PID. Though PID is often bilateral, this is not always true, and the pain of appendicitis can present in an atypical position, including bilaterally. Overlapping symptoms make mistakes in preoperative diagnosis inevitable. If more than 80 percent of exploratory laparotomies are confirming acute appendicitis, it may mean that surgery is being delayed too long. Since 10 percent of patients may have pyuria or microscopic hematuria, it occasionally may be difficult to differentiate acute appendicitis from severe cystitis or renal colic.

Liberal use of the laparoscope has been advocated by Jacobson and Westrum to confirm all cases of PID. The inflammed appendix usually can be seen through the laparoscope. An aggressive diagnostic approach is indicated in those patients presumed to have PID who do not readily respond to antibiotics. Those with gonorrheal salpingitis should show clinical improvement within 24 hours of antibiotics.

If salpingitis is noted at laparotomy, the pelvic organs should not be manipulated. Aggressive parenteral antibiotics should be begun, usually penicillin and an aminoglycoside or also clindamycin. A gram stain and aerobic and anaerobic culture of the cul-de-sac fluid may help determine antibiotic coverage.

In children, the differential diagnosis includes no organ pathology, acute mesenteric lymphadenitis, acute gastroenteritis, acute pyelonephritis, Meckel's diverticulitis, intussusception, regional enteritis, primary peritonitis, and Henoch-Schönlein purpura.

In mesenteric adenitis, there is usually a recent upper respiratory infection, and the pain and tenderness is not as specific as appendicitis. There also may be generalized lymphadenopathy. Close observation in the hospital may occasionally differentiate the two. Of course, in gastroenteritis, diarrhea is usually a more prominent finding, and there is less discomfort with movement and ambulation. Intussusception is more common under the age of two, and is characterized by episodic colicky pain with intermittent well-being. It can be treated with a therapeutic barium enema, which should be avoided in appendicitis. Pain medications and laxatives need to be withheld when appendicitis is being considered.

Regional enteritis may present with fever, right lower quadrant pain and tenderness, and leukocytosis. Diarrhea is more common and anorexia less common than in appendicitis. Frequently, the diagnosis of regional enteritis is first made at exploratory laparotomy for pelvic pain.

Diverticula of the sigmoid colon are common in older women. When these diverticulum become inflamed, they can present with symptoms and signs very similar to appendicitis or PID. Usually there is left lower quadrant pain, constipation, and nausea. A low grade fever with left lower quadrant tenderness and guarding occurs with a leukocytosis. The pain is usually described as dull, aching, and constant. Differential diagnosis includes carcinoma of the bowel. Sigmoidoscopy should be done early in the course and barium enema performed after the acute stage. Initial therapy is conservative with nasogastric suction, parenteral fluids and antibiotics. If no improvement occurs, then surgery is indicated.

REFERENCES

1. Marshall WA and Tanner JM: Variation in pattern of pubertal changes in girls. Arch Dis Child 44:291, 1969.
2. Mishell Jr DR: Assessing the intrauterine device. Fam Plan Perspect 7:103, 1975.
3. Wilson RT and Ledger WJ: Complications associated with the intrauterine contraceptive device in women of middle and upper socioeconomic class. Am J Obstet Gynecol 100:649, 1968.

4. Wright NH and Laemmle P: Acute pelvic inflammatory disease in an indigent population. An estimate of its incidence and relationship to method of contraception. Am J Obstet Gynecol, 101:979, 1968.
5. Cates Jr W, et al: The intrauterine device and,deaths from spontaneous abortion. N Engl J Med 295:1155, 1976.
6. Taylor ES, et al: The intrauterine device and tubo-ovarian abscess. Am J Obstet Gynecol 123:338, 1975.
7. Bukovsky I, et al: Conservative surgery for tubal pregnancy. Obstet Gynecol 53:709, 1979.
8. Schoen J and Nowak RJ: Repeat ectopic pregnancy. Obstet Gynecol 45:542, 1975.
9. Breen JL: A 21 year survey of 654 ectopic pregnancies. Am J Obstet Gynecol 106:1004, 1970.
10. Westrum L: Effects of acute pelvic inflammatory disease on fertility. Am J Obstet Gynecol 121:707, 1975.
11. Schaefer G: Tuberculosis of the female genital tract. Clin Obstet Gynecol 13:965, 1970.
12. Wolf G and Thompson N: Female sterilization and subsequent ectopic pregnancy. Obstet Gynecol 55:17, 1980.
13. Brenner PF, Benedetti T, and Mishall Jr DR: Ectopic pregnancy following tubal sterilization surgery. Obstet Gynecol 49:323, 1977.
14. Ory HW: Ectopic pregnancy and intrauterine contraceptive devices: new perspectives. Personal communication. The Women's Health Study, Center for Disease Control, Atlanta.
15. Berry CM, Thompson JD, and Hatcher R: The radioreceptor assay for HCG in ectopic pregnancy. Obstet Gynecol 54:43, 1979.
16. Schoenbaum S, et al: Gray-scale ultrasound in tubal pregnancy. Radiology 127:757, 1978.
17. Kelly MT, et al: The value of sonography in suspected ectopic pregnancy. Obstet Gynecol 53:703, 1979.
18. Novak E and Woodruff JR: Gynecologic and Obstetric Pathology. W.B. Saunders. Philadelphia, 1974.
19. Eriksen P and Philipsen T: Prognosis on threatened abortion evaluated by hormone assays and ultrasound scanning. Obstet Gynecol 55:435, 1980.
20. Ominsky A: Blood transfusion and intravenous technique. In Dripps R, Eckenhoff J and Vandam L, Eds: Introduction to Anesthesia. 4th Ed. W.B. Saunders, Philadelphia, 1972.
21. ACOG Technical Bulletin #50, June 1978: Sexually transmitted diseases. The American College of Obstetricians and Gynecologists, Chicago.
22. Handsfield HH, et al: Asymptomatic gonorrhea in men. N Engl J Med 290:117, 1974.
23. Eschenbach DA and Holmes K: Acute pelvic inflammatory disease: current concepts of pathogenesis, etiology, and management. Clin Obstet Gynecol, 18: 1974.
24. Mardh PA, et al: Chlamydin Trachomatis infection in patients with acute salpingitis. N Engl J Med 296:24, 1977.
25. Jacobson L and Westrum L: Objectivized diagnosis of acute pelvic inflammatory disease. Am J Obstet Gynecol 105:1088, 1969.
26. Falk V: Treatment of acute non-tuberculous salpingitis with antibiotics alone and in combination with glucocorticords. Acta Obstet Gynecol Scand (Suppl) 44:65, 1965.
27. Cunningham FG, et al: Evaluation of tetracycline or penicillin and ampicillin for treatment of acute pelvic inflammatory disease. N Engl J Med 296:24, 1977.

28. Center for Disease Control Recommended Treatment Schedules, 1979: Gonorrhea. Ann Intern Med 90:809, 1979.
29. Lee RA and Welch J: Torsion of the uterine adnexa. Am J Obstet Gynecol 97:974, 1967.
30. Dresler S: Antenatal torsion of a normal ovary and fallopian tube. Am J Dis Child 131: 1977.
31. Powell J, et al: Torsion of the fallopian tube in postmenopausal women. Am J Obstet Gynecol 113:236, 1977.
32. Storer E: Appendix. In Schwartz, Seymour, et al, Eds: Principles of Surgery. McGraw-Hill, 1979.

7 Abnormal Vaginal Bleeding

Gilbert G. Haas, Jr.

An emergency room physician may be called upon both to provide care for women with massive amounts of vaginal hemorrhage and also for women with less dramatic abnormal bleeding. At such times, he must be able to differentiate an isolated episode of abnormal bleeding from similar bleeding secondary to an undiagnosed long-term disease process. Any vaginal bleeding that appears at an unexpected time or in an unexpected amount should be considered abnormal. A woman's reproductive life spans the ages from 10 to 50, and bleeding in any amount before or after this interval is considered abnormal and demands further evaluation. Following the menarche, any bleeding that occurs outside a woman's regular menstrual pattern is also suspect, although most women have occasional anovulatory cycles that can either lengthen or shorten the interval between bleeding episodes.

The average menstrual flow occurs every 28 days, although regular patterns of bleeding that occur every 25 to 32 days should probably also be considered normal.[1] The majority of menses last from 1 to 8 days; [1] longer bleeding episodes can be an additional cause for concern. Although many women profess to a clock-like accuracy to their menstrual pattern, cycle-to-cycle variations do occur for a plethora of reasons, including anovulation, increasing age, acute stress, or changes that follow a pregnancy. These diagnoses must be sorted from the more ominous ones that could result in long-term harm to the patient's health.

VAGINAL BLEEDING IN THE VERY YOUNG PATIENT (UNDER AGE 10)

The amount of vaginal bleeding in patients of this age group will only rarely be of sufficient quantity to disturb physiological function. However, the younger patient and her parents will frequently express a greater degree of concern than that found in older patients who experience far greater amounts of blood loss. Therefore, it is of prime importance to consider these fears and concerns in the approach to the young patient and her problem.

The majority of vaginal bleeding in the prepubertal female is associated with precocious puberty.[2] Other causes of genital bleeding in this age group include genital tumor (12 percent), trauma (8 percent), vaginitis (6 percent), and vaginal prolapse (2 percent) (Table 7.1). The major obstacle to a correct diagnosis is the inability to perform a pelvic examination properly because of one or more of the following factors: lack of patient cooperation; improper instrumentation; failure of the patient's parents to understand the necessity of a pelvic examination; failure of the physician to exhibit the herculean patience necessary to examine successfully these young patients.

Hormonally active ovarian tumors may cause irregular vaginal bleeding, which at times may be heavy in amount.[3] Most of these tumors may be palpated during a single-digit rectal examination. Frequently, this can be painlessly performed, particularly if the proposed examination is explained adequately to the patient in terms that she can understand. The diagnosis of sarcoma botryoides is frequently delayed because of its deceptively benign gross or even microscopic appearance.[4] Until recently, adenocarcinomas of the vagina and cervix were considered rare in this age group. However, since the report of Herbst et al,[5] the mother should be questioned about stilbestrol (DES) or other estrogen ingestion early in her pregnancy if her daughter presents with vaginal bleeding. The problem is complicated by the fact that as many as one-fourth of the mothers whose daughters have carcinoma of the vagina did not take DES.[5] Vaginal bleeding that is thought secondary to sexual assault or blunt trauma warrants examination under anesthesia to document thoroughly the extent of the injury. In cases of suspected sexual assault, an attempt should also be made to identify sperm, acid phosphatase, or other incriminating evidence within the vagina.

Vulvovaginitis can occasionally cause small amounts of bleeding.[2] In the author's experience, bleeding is more frequently associated with monilial vaginitis than with vaginitis of bacterial or trichomonal etiology. The latter protozoa occurs very rarely in the unestrogenized vaginas of prepubertal females.[2] The diagnosis can be made by either selective culture or microscopic examina-

Table 7-1. Causes of vaginal bleeding in the prepubertal female.

Precocious puberty
Genital tumor
Trauma
Vaginitis
Vaginal prolapse

tion of the vaginal discharge. A sample of discharge can frequently be collected by simply inserting a moistened cotton applicator through the gently spread labia. Ten percent potassium hydroxide (KOH) can be added to the drop of vaginal secretions to lyse the epithelial and blood cells, but leave the Candida hyphae intact for easier identification. A frequently associated finding, particularly if the infection is associated with bleeding, is a reddened, excoriated vulva, with a history of incessant scratching in the genital area. Healing of such lesions is speeded by the application of a cream containing both a moniliocidal agent and a corticosteroid (Mycolog).

Monilial vaginitis is treated by local therapy for about one week. A 20 cc syringe with a 14 gauge plastic intravenous catheter is given to the parents in the emergency room and is filled with a moniliocidal agent and refrigerated. The parents can then safely insert 1 to 2 cc of the medication at bedtime through the small catheter into the child's vagina with minimal, if any pain. The parents should also apply a small amount of the drug to the child's labia and vulva to relieve the pruritus in these areas.

Bacterial infections can occur in children, particularly after they have assumed responsibility for their toilet habits. Such infections are only occasionally associated with vaginal bleeding, usually noticed when a spot or two of blood appears on the young patient's panties. Bacterial infections are best treated with systemic therapy.[6] The choice of drug depends upon the results of culture and sensitivity of the vaginal discharge. Tetracycline should be avoided in this age group because it can cause staining of the tooth enamel. A suspension of ampicillin for 1 week in the lower dosage ranges usually suffices, since the majority of infections are secondary to colonic organisms sensitive to this antibiotic.[7] The patient's toilet habits should be closely monitored to insure that further vaginal contamination from the perianal area does not occur.

Patients suspected of having precocious puberty should either be immediately admitted for endocrine, roentgenographic, or genetic testing; or referred to a physician interested in and capable of treating this type of problem. Precocious puberty can be divided into complete and incomplete forms. The latter is defined as the appearance of an isolated pubertal change (breast development, pubic hair, or axillary hair) without any of the other effects of estrogen, such as vaginal bleeding.

Complete isosexual precocious puberty can be subdivided into true and pseudoisosexual forms. Ninety percent of all female patients with complete isosexual precocious puberty will have the true form. In these cases, a normal sequence of pubertal events occurs at an early age. Ninety percent (81 percent of the total) of these female patients with true isosexual precocious puberty have constitutional or idiopathic disease, often complicated by the psychologic trauma inflicted by the young girl's peers.[8] At first, these patients are much taller than their friends, but ultimately they will be very short in stature because of premature epiphyseal closure. The earlier the disease begins, the shorter will be the patient's final height. Fifty percent have EEG abnormalities consistent with epilepsy. Although the onset of symptoms can occur at any age, they are rare in the first year of life. The remaining patients with true isosexual precocious puberty have organic brain disease, caused by tumors, congenital defects, obstructive processes, or postinfective lesions, usually involving the hypothalmus, which results in neurologic signs and symptoms.

In the young patients with pseudoisosexual precocious puberty, development of secondary sex characteristics is not accompanied by proper cyclic function of the hypothalamic-pituitary-ovarian axis. These patients can have one of six disease entities: (1) estrogen-secreting ovarian tumors, especially of the granulosa-theca cell type (Sufficient treatment is usually unilateral oophorectomy, since most tumors are benign.); (2) the very rare estrogen-secreting adrenal tumors; (3) iatrogenic causes secondary to the oral or topical administration of estrogens (A detailed history is the key to this diagnosis.); (4) hypothyroidism, which can cause a concomitant increase in gonadotropins in parallel with thyroid stimulating hormone (TSH); (5) the McCune-Albright syndrome—the combination of sexual precocity, multiple areas of fibrous or cystic dysplasia of the bone, and brown or cafe-au-lait spots on the skin, usually occurring after 2 years of age; and (6) hemihypertrophy—a rare combination of unilateral sexual precocity associated with various vascular anomalies.[8]

In making the diagnosis, the patient's bone age should be evaluated first. Hypothyroid patients will have a retarded bone age, while a bone age in agreement with the chronologic age suggests the incomplete form of precocious puberty. The advancement of bone age above the 95th percentile indicates a peripheral estrogen effect. Gonadotropins are increased in the true forms of sexual precocity, while depressed in the pseudo forms.

Since 90 percent of all girls with isosexual precocious puberty have constitutional precocity, the ideal therapy would result in regression of the secondary sex characteristics, would prevent the accelerated growth and premature fusion of the distal epiphyses, cause cessation of menstruation, and prevent fertility. Medroxyprogesterone acetate, danazol, and cyproterone acetate have all been used, the former most frequently. None has achieved totally satisfactory results.

Patients in this age group in whom the etiology of their vaginal bleeding is not clear, or on whom it is not possible to carry out a pelvic examination, should be referred for urological or gynecological consultation. Vaginoscopy, laparoscopy, or other tests are necessary in these patients to rule out a foreign body or a lesion hidden within the vagina.

BLEEDING IN THE REPRODUCTIVE AGE GROUP (AGES 10 TO 35)

In the first year following the menarche, up to 55 percent of a young girl's bleeding episodes are not preceded by ovulation. As a result, it takes about 15 months to complete the first 10 menstrual cycles. This percentage of anovulatory cycles decreases until at gynecological age 8 only 5 to 10 percent of the bleeding episodes are anovulatory.[9] At the time of menarche, the release of gonadotropin stimulates the ovary to produce estrogen. Ovulation, however, cannot occur until the hypothalamic-pituitary-ovarian axis matures, and the positive feedback mechanism to rising levels of estrogen is established. Until regular ovulation begins, unopposed estrogen results in continuous proliferation of the endometrium. The amount of proliferation and the stability of the endometrium depends upon the level of estrogen that is present. When the estrogen level falls below a critical threshold level, uterine bleeding occurs. This threshold is determined both by the amount of estrogen that is present, and the degree of endometrial proliferation that has occurred.

If estrogen levels are very high and then fall precipitously, the bleeding that results stems from inefficient shedding of a thickened endometrium, and the menses may be prolonged and profuse. High estrogen levels can also result in a hyperplastic endometrium that outgrows the amount of estrogen support that is available to it. Low estrogen levels cause a more gradual proliferation, and oligomenorrhea may result. If the level of estrogen approximates the threshold value needed to sustain endometrial integrity, spotting can appear whenever the estrogen level dips below the threshold value. Finally, if prolonged bleeding occurs, portions of the basal endometriun can be lost, exposing large myometrial arterioles which can profusely hemorrhage.[10]

Thus, in the young post-menarchal female, abnormal bleeding can range from a few cycles of irregular bleeding, to almost continuous spotting, to major hemorrhage. The patient's history, physical examination, and initial laboratory studies should alert the emergency room physician to the particular systemic or structural lesion causing the abnormal bleeding episode. Even though the majority of such bleeding will be secondary to post-menarchal anovulation, an index of suspicion should always be maintained for other conditions that might result in vaginal bleeding in this age group. Physical examination should concentrate on several points, including signs of central nervous system lesions, an enlarged thyroid gland, expressible galactorrhea, palpable abdominal masses, and any abnormality of the pelvic examination. Both a speculum and a bimanual examination should be performed to locate the exact source of the bleeding. Even in the younger, virginal patient, a thorough examination is possible if sufficient explanation is given, and a small speculum is used. If an examination is impossible, or in those cases in which an anatomical abnormality is suggested, examination under anesthesia should be strongly considered.

Since anovulation is not the only cause of vaginal bleeding in the young female, other etiologies should be suspected (Table 7.2). These include:

1. *Complications of pregnancy*. Ectopic gestation, spontaneous abortion, hydatidiform mole, or other vaginal bleeding secondary to an abnormality of a pregnancy. If the sexual history, prior menstrual pattern, and the presence of morning nausea, fatigue, or other subjective signs of pregnancy suggest this as a possibility, a pregnancy test should be performed. Using the sensitive serum tests for circulating chorionic gonadotropin, early pregnancies, ectopic gestations, or threatened abortions can be diagnosed.[11] If a quantitative test is available, a very high level would suggest a molar gestation.

Table 7-2. Causes of bleeding in the reproductive age group.

Anovulatory bleeding
Complications of pregnancy
Anatomic abnormalities
Abnormalities of other endocrine systems
Coagulation defects
Female hyperandrogenism
Miscellaneous factors

2. *Anatomic abnormalities.*

A. Benign: Cervical polyps, cervicitis, endometrial polyps, leiomyomas, pelvic inflammation, or vaginal adenosis secondary to prenatal stilbestrol exposure.

B. Malignant: Leukemia, trophoblastic disease, carcinomas, sarcomas, or similar lesions that may rarely occur in this age group.

3. *Abnormalities of other endocrine systems.* Hypo- or hyperthyroidism, adrenal disorders, or diabetes are only rarely diagnosed. If thyroid dysfunction is suggested, a TSH determination should be included along with any thyroid function testing to rule out minimal abnormalities and help determine the site of endocrine malfunction.

4. *Coagulation defects.* Prothrombin time, partial thromboplastin time, and a platelet count should be ordered.

5. *Female hyperandrogenism:* polycystic ovarian disease (PCOD or Stein-Leventhal syndrome). Plasma testosterone, free testosterone, and dehydroepiandrosterone sulfate level may diagnose the abnormality and suggest the site of increased androgenic secretion.[12]

6. *Miscellaneous factors.* Obesity, drug abuse, or emotional disturbances.

The appropriate laboratory tests should be ordered to screen patients for these disorders. Coagulation testing and a platelet count can document the adequacy of the clotting mechanism. A complete blood count will determine the effect of blood loss on the patient's red blood cell mass and document the normalcy of the patient's leukocytes. A serum pregnancy test should be requested, particularly if the patient admits to sexual activity and is not using contraceptives. Other endocrine testing should be considered, but these tests are usually helpful only if the history or physical examination suggests a particular dysfunction. In some patients, basal temperature monitoring might be appropriate to determine if ovulation, oligo-ovulation, or anovulation is present. Temperatures should be recorded each morning between two consecutive bleeding episodes. A prolactin determination is only rarely elevated in patients with excessive bleeding. However, if galactorrhea is present, or if the interval between oligomenorrheic bleeding episodes is increasing, then such testing is appropriate.[13]

Anovulatory Bleeding

In a young woman, anovulatory bleeding and secondary endometrial hyperplasia is a potential problem.[14] In an ovulatory cycle, menses follow progesterone induction of a structurally stable secretory endometrium. With regression of the corpus luteum, there is a sudden decrease of ovarian steroids, in particular progesterone, that results in spasm of the endometrial spiral arterioles. Because of the decreased blood flow, endometrial ischemia and necrosis occurs, and the outer layers of the endometrium are sloughed in a uniform fashion. The onset and cessation of the bleeding is usually abrupt. In the patient with chronic anovulation, unopposed estrogen stimulation is continuous. Endometrial hyperplasia and possible endometrial carcinoma may occur even in a young patient following several months or years of continuous estrogen stimulation. As a result, the physician must not only control the acute bleeding episode, but also consider the long-term consequences of unopposed estrogen upon the endometrium.

In the young adolescent patient, small amounts of irregular bleeding for only a few months are best managed by simple observation. The patient and her parents are advised of the necessity of followup and should be reassured that hematologic testing has shown that the blood loss has had no effect upon the patient's red blood cell mass. Furthermore, they should be told that a daughter may not mirror the early menstrual history of her mother.

In the somewhat older patient with several years of menstrual irregularity, the patient's followup should be supervised by a physician interested in and capable of handling such problems. Although oral contraceptives are frequently prescribed for these young women to "regulate their periods," time will cure the majority of short-term bleeding irregularity, and hypothalamic suppression by oral contraceptives may only aggravate an already suppressed hypothalamic-ovarian axis. In a patient in this age group, it is most appropriate to make a diagnosis of the cause of the abnormal bleeding before therapeutic maneuvers are begun. At the very least plasma samples should be drawn, refrigerated, and reserved for later testing if warranted. Cyclical progestational agents or oral contraceptives as a progestin source may eventually be indicated, but these medications should be administered only to treat a known malady and not used as a "shot in the dark" panacea for the problem. If the patient is to be referred to a reproductive endocrinologist, time can be saved by ordering the appropriate laboratory studies or at least collecting pre-treatment plasmas during the patient's emergency room visit.

When a woman is seen in an emergency room for abnormal vaginal bleeding, she can be placed into one of two categories based upon the degree of blood loss present. Patients with minor amounts of bleeding should be advised of the proper diagnostic maneuvers they should undergo, particularly if the abnormal bleeding has occurred over a prolonged time interval. As mentioned, in the younger, post-menarchal patient, watchful waiting is the best course unless the blood loss is severe. In the older patient with mild to moderate vaginal bleeding, diagnostic blood samples can be obtained, and then hemostasis achieved with either intramuscular (IM) or oral progestational agents. When anovulatory vaginal bleeding occurs, the ovaries are not providing their own stabilizing progesterone following ovulation, and an exogenous progestational agent—progesterone in oil, 100 to 200 mg IM; medroxyprogesterone acetate (Provera), 10 mg po qd × 5 days; or norethindrone (Norlutin), 10 mg po qd × 5 days—must be given. However, continuous bleeding over a long interval of time can strip the uterus of all endometrium. If no endometrium is present for progesterone to influence, hemostasis cannot be obtained when only a progestational agent is prescribed. In such cases, estrogen must also be given to effect endometrial growth so that tissue is available upon which the progestational agent can act.

Endometrial curettage is a diagnostic, not a therapeutic procedure. In this age group, a uterine curettage is usually unnecessary for diagnosis because of the minimal risk of malignancy. Furthermore, the successful treatment of the majority of these patients with a chemical hormonal curettage obviates the need for a surgical or anesthetic risk. Curettage is reserved for bleeding unresponsive to hormonal therapy, recurrent severe bleeding, or when the suspicion of endometrial hyperplasia or another anatomic lesion exists. Nevertheless, mothers are eager to recall "cures" either they or close friends have experienced following a uterine curettage for abnormal bleeding. They should be reminded of the risks involved during general anesthesia (cardio-pulmonary collapse) and surgical manipulation (uterine perforation), of the possible effects of dilation and curettage on subsequent fertility (Asherman's syndrome or cervical incompetence), of the risk of post-operative endometritis, and, perhaps most importantly, of the fact that the young patient's bleeding problem may quickly recur, unlike the case of the woman in whom a one-time anovulatory cycle was successfully "cured" by a D&C. Moreover, prior to the availability of oral progestin therapy, hormonal therapy was not available, and this may have been the reason for surgical intervention.

If the bleeding is so severe that it warrants hospitalization for blood volume replacement and rapid hemostasis, either oral or intravenous estrogenic and progestational agents can be used. Reasons for choosing parenteral therapy include: (1) severe bleeding requiring rapid hemostasis, (2) the failure of oral agents to control the bleeding, and (3) persistent and incessant vomiting secondary to estrogen administration with possible failure of drug absorption.

Twenty-five mg of conjugated estrogen (Premarin) can be administered intravenously every 2 to 6 hours until the bleeding is controlled. If the bleeding is not controlled within a 12-hour timespan, then the diagnosis of dysfunctional bleeding should be re-evaluated. Oral or intramuscular estrogens can also be used. High-dose, orally-administered estrogen, equivalent to 2.5 to 5 mg of conjugated estrogens, should initially be given 4 times a day. Alternatively, 250 mg of intramuscular estradiol valerate (Delestrogen) are particularly appropriate when there is gastrointestinal intolerance to orally-administered estrogens. Another possibility is to begin a high-dose oral estrogen/progestin combination, such as norethynodrel 5 or 10 mg with mestranol 0.075 mg (Enovid 5 or 10 mg), 4 times a day. An antiemetic may be necessary because of the nausea and vomiting produced by the estrogen in any of these regimens. The combination pill produces both endometrial build-up by estrogenic stimulation and rapid conversion to secretory endometrium by the progestational agent. If estrogen alone is used initially to control the uterine bleeding, the endometrium should be stabilized by the administration of a progestational agent. Medroxyprogesterone acetate or norethindrone can be given in doses of 10 to 20 mg daily for the last 7 to 10 days of estrogen administration; the estrogen is given for a total of 2 to 3 weeks. Medroxyprogesterone acetate is not thought to be a totally effective hemostatic agent when it is used alone.[9] If patient compliance is doubtful, hemostasis can be obtained with estrogenic drugs, and then 250 mg of hydroxyprogesterone caproate (Delalutin) can be given concomitantly with either an injection of estradiol valerate, or the continuation of oral estrogens for 2 more weeks. In either case, vaginal bleeding should be expected 2 weeks after the intramuscular progestational agent has been given. A combination of estrogen/progestin should be continued for 2 to 3 cycles after the bleeding is brought under control. This is most easily accomplished by administering an oral contraceptive agent. Many women are relieved to have an interval free of abnormal vaginal bleeding caused by the vicious cycle of continued anovulation and further bleeding. If the amount of bleeding has decreased the red blood cell count, vitamins containing folic acid and iron can be prescribed (Table 7.3).

Moderate amounts of vaginal bleeding do not necessitate hospitalization, since out-patient stabilization of the endometrium can be achieved with high-dose estrogen/progestin combinations given intramuscularly or orally, either in a sequential or a combined form. If oral therapy is chosen, an estrogen/progestin combination can be given 4 times a day until the bleeding is controlled. The number of daily doses are then decreased while continuing to monitor the amount of blood loss. Norethynodrel 5 mg with mestranol 0.075 mg (Enovid 5 mg) is an effective agent for this purpose.

When the endometrium has successfully stabilized on one tablet per day, this dosage is continued for 2 to 3 additional weeks to assure an interval free of blood loss. Breakthrough bleeding can be managed by administering small amounts of additional estrogen (equivalent to 0.6 to 1.25 mg of conjugated estrogen per day) for a few days. The patient or her parents should be warned that a bleeding episode, possibly with cramping, will begin when the drug is discontinued. The dysmenorrhea can be alleviated by one of the prostaglandin synthetase inhibitors, such as ibuprofen (Motrin) 400 mg 3 to 4 times per day, or mefenamic acid (Ponstel) 250 mg every 6 hours.[15] Just as the patient who must be hospitalized, the woman treated as an out-patient should also continue 2 to 3 months on an estrogen/progestin combination to assure an interval of controlled vaginal bleeding. If the amount of bleeding during the initial progestational withdrawal is only mild or moderate, the second cycle of medication is begun on day 5 to 7 of the cycle. If heavy withdrawal bleeding occurs, the

Table 7-3. Treatment of severe vaginal bleeding.

1. Conjugated estrogens (Premarin) 25 mg IV q 2–6 hr., followed by
2. High dose estrogens po (Premarin 5 mg qd) Followed by
3. Cyclic estrogen/progestin therapy for 2–3 months.

medication can be begun earlier in the cycle, around day 2 or 3, to help control excessive menorrhagia. Although the patient or her parents should definitely be warned of the possible side effects of estrogen-containing medications, the relative risk of the medication should be compared to the risk of surgical intervention, rather than against the risk of other methods of contraception, the comparison the patient or her parents will probably make using the information available to them in the lay press.

In the case of the woman who is suspected of having had a single anovulatory cycle and is experiencing bleeding that is abnormal only in its timing, but not its amount, intramuscular progesterone in oil (100 to 200 mg IM) is an effective agent to transform the endometrium to the secretory type and effect a withdrawal bleeding episode once the administered drug level has dissipated. The patient should be warned that although the present bleeding episode will stop, she should expect a second menstrual flow within a week after the administration of the drug. Another option in these cases is to administer a single package of oral contraceptives at the usual one pill a day dosage.

Hyperandrogenism

If the patient is not hospitalized, arrangements should be made to diagnose the cause of the abnormal bleeding rather than only treating the symptomatology without further diagnosis. In a considerable number of women of reproductive age, hyperandrogenism can be associated with anovulatory cycles. In fact, it has been cited as the most frequent hormonal abnormality in women.[16] The telltale symptoms of hirsutism, acne, bilaterally enlarged ovaries, and irregular menstrual bleeding imply the diagnosis. The amount of hirsutism does not have to be extreme to warrant investigation of the patient's circulating androgen levels in the form of testosterone, free testosterone, and dehydroepiandrosterone sulfate. Testosterone can be produced by either the ovary or the adrenal gland, while dehydroepiandrosterone sulfate is almost totally produced by the adrenal gland.[17] Following initial laboratory testing, the patient should be referred to a reproductive endocrinologist for therapy. Circulating androgen levels should be determined in women with a prolonged history of abnormal menstrual bleeding. Plasma for later studies should be drawn prior to the administration of any estrogen/progestin combination since the ovarian suppression that occurs secondary to these drugs may invalidate circulating androgen evaluation for some time.

If the diagnosis of female hyperandrogenism is made, subsequent therapy will depend on the answers to two questions. The first is: does the patient desire a pregnancy at the present time? If the answer is affirmative, an ovulation induction agent, such as clomiphene, can be begun (50 to 100 mg a day for 5 days beginning on day 5 of the woman's cycle). If the hyperandrogenism originates from the adrenal gland, as manifested by an elevated dehydroepiandrosterone sulfate level, ovulation can frequently be induced following adrenal suppression with exogenously administered, low-dose corticosteroids. A 2-week trial of maximal dexamethasone suppression (dexamethasone, 0.5 mg po 4 times a day) is followed by a second determination of the plasma androgen levels.[18] Although glucocorticoid secretion by the adrenal gland can be suppressed by a single dose of exogenous corticosteroids, adrenal suppression frequently requires a much longer period of time.[19] While awaiting the second set of laboratory results, the patient is continued on a lowered dose of dexamethasone each night. The late evening dosage maximally suppresses the early morning peak in the adrenal circadian cycle. If there is no suppression of the androgen levels, the corticosteroids are discontinued, and clomiphene is begun to effect ovulation. If, on the other hand, the androgens have been suppressed, the single nighttime dose is continued, and the possible onset of ovulation is monitored by recording the patient's morning basal temperature curve. Ovulation will frequently occur within 1 to 4 months while on this regimen.[20] If ovulation does not occur, a third androgen determination should be obtained to compare the degree of adrenal suppression with the lowered corticosteroid dosage (0.5 mg po qd) to that seen with maximal suppression (dexamethasone 0.5 mg po qid). If comparable androgen suppression has not occurred with the lower dosage, the corticosteroid can be increased by adding 0.25 mg of dexamethasone each morning. Symptoms of Cushing's disease should be watched for, although even with the increased dosage, this occurs infrequently. If anovulation continues despite adequate androgen suppression, clomiphene should be administered while continuing the androgen suppression. If elevated circulating androgen levels are suppressed, the dosage of clomiphene is frequently less than that previously necessary to effect ovulation.

If the patient does not desire childbearing at the present time, the second question to be asked is: does the patient have signs of hyperandrogenism, such as acne or hirsutism? In patients with these complaints, particularly if they are progressive, ovarian or adrenal suppression should be performed, if only to document the suppressibility of the androgen production and to rule out (to a degree) adrenal or ovarian tumors. Very high androgen levels, regardless of their suppressibility, suggest the presence of a hormonally-active tumor.[21] The patient with mild hirsutism should be advised that the condition can be progressive. Although when the elevated androgen levels are lowered, in many patients there is no further progression of the amount of hair growth, frequently no regression occurs, and the best that can be hoped for is stabilization at the present level of hirsutism.[22] The patient should be counseled that although there may be rapid relief of the problem of acne, it may take as long as 4 to 6 months of suppression before there is a noticeable reduction or change in the masculine pattern of hair growth.[23] The delay is perhaps due to the necessity of the coarse hair, formed when the androgen levels were elevated, to be pushed from the follicle in due course. Electrolysis in patients who have little regression of hair growth is a much more effective therapeutic adjuvant following adequate suppression of elevated androgen levels. Frequently, one of the first signs noted by the patient already undergoing electrolysis will be a decreased number of electrolysis appointments necessary to achieve satisfactory cosmetic results.

The protocol for adrenal suppression has been described. For ovarian suppression, 2 mg of norethindrone and 0.1 mg of mestranol (Ortho-Novum or Norinyl 2 mg) has been shown to be the estrogen/progestin combination that achieves the lowest free, non-protein-bound androgen level.[24] If there is a contraindication to the administration of such high levels of estrogen, then one of the other oral contraceptives containing less estrogen can be tried, although in some patients less satisfactory results may be obtained. Occasionally such a patient will respond to one, but not another estrogen/progestin combination, depending on the estrogenic strength of the progestational agent in the oral contraceptive. As with adrenal suppression, the results of ovarian suppression are monitored with a second plasma sample to determine if the androgen levels have been suppressed after 1 month of medication. If suppression is successful, it is sometimes possible to lower the dosage of estrogen to 0.080 or 0.050 mg of mestranol (Ortho-Novum or Norinyl 1/80 or 1/50 respectively), and achieve satisfactory results. The subjective symptoms of the patient and the results of further androgen testing should be closely monitored, as some patients require resumption of the higher estrogen dose. For economic reasons, the adequacy of ovarian or adrenal suppression can frequently be monitored by the patient's subjective appraisal of her symptoms, or a single androgen level can be determined, i.e., testosterone or dehydroepiandrosterone sulfate, the choice depending upon which hormone demonstrated the greatest elevation prior to therapy.

Suppression and stimulation testing has failed in many cases to pinpoint adequately the site of androgen over-production.[25] An elevated dehydroepiandrosterone sulfate level suggests an adrenal source, but increased testosterone production can occur in either the ovary or the adrenal gland. Because of this dilemma, a target gland to be suppressed is chosen initially, and the results of therapy must be monitored to determine the correctness of the choice. In the case of ovarian suppression, oral contraceptives are given for a specific medical indication, not to "kill two birds with one stone" because they also supply contraception. An oral contraceptive is chosen for ovarian suppression because of the convenience of taking a single tablet containing both estrogen and progestin. This results in ovarian suppression while maintaining the stability of the endometrium with minimal breakthrough bleeding. The effective contraception that ensues should be thought of as a side effect, perhaps desired by the patient, but it is not the prime reason for the choice of ovarian suppression therapy. However, the desire on the patient's part for effective contraception may guide the physician as to which gland, the ovary or the adrenal, undergoes an initial trial of suppression when the correct choice is not clear following initial androgen testing. Successful androgen suppression can occur with dexamethasone, even if the dehydroepiandrosterone sulfate level is normal, if there is an elevated production of testosterone from an adrenal source. This becomes particularly important in the older patient with abnormal uterine bleeding thought to be due to anovulation secondary to hyperandrogenism, since, in this age group, there is an increased risk of estrogenic side effects. Successful androgen suppression following corticosteroid administration is even more likely to occur in patients with an elevated dehydroepiandrosterone sulfate level. In a few patients, both ovarian and adrenal suppression is necessary to achieve adequate androgen suppression and relief of symptoms. In some patients with symptoms apparently due to hyperandrogenism, normal androgen levels are found. In many of these patients, the lowering of the androgen levels following suppression therapy is associated with relief of their symptomatology. These patients are thought to have an increased sensitivity of their hair follicles to "normal" levels of androgens.[22]

If treatment failure occurs, either because of a lack of relief of symptoms or because of inadequate biochemical suppression, then the target of hormonal suppression should be re-evaluated and possibly altered. It must be remembered, in the case of dexamethasone suppression, that even if the androgen levels are satisfactorily suppressed, yet ovulation does not subsequently occur, an exogenous progestational agent should be given every 5 to 8 weeks to prevent endometrial hyperplasia secondary to unopposed estrogen stimulation.

If no subjective symptoms of hyperandrogenism are present, then the patient should be encouraged to employ cyclically a progestational agent to prevent endometrial hyperplasia and the possibility of subsequent endometrial malignancy. The patient may take an oral contraceptive or a progestational agent alone. In the former case, any oral contraceptive may be chosen, since androgenic suppression is not a consideration. Oral progestins (medroxyprogesterone acetate, 10 mg, or norlutin, 10 mg) can be given for 5 days every 5 to 8 weeks without estrogenic side effects. These drugs are not administered more frequently because they could mask the return of spontaneous ovulation. If spontaneous bleeding occurs between the progestational withdrawal bleeding episodes, or if no withdrawal bleeding occurs when the progestin is administered, then the medication should be discontinued temporarily. The possible return of spontaneous ovulatory function (documented by basal temperature monitoring) or the presence of a pregnancy (manifested by a positive serum pregnancy test) should be sought. If anovulation is still present, then the interval between progestin administration should be shortened to prevent further breakthrough bleeding. If, on the other hand, failure of withdrawal occurs, but a pregnancy is not present, then the cause of such progestin withdrawal should be sought by monitoring estrogen, gonadotropin, and prolactin levels (to rule out a lowered secretion of estrogen by the ovary, ovarian failure manifested by an elevation of pituitary gonadotropins, or hyperprolatinemia, respectively). The possibility of endometrial damage from an overzealous D&C should also be considered and can be diagnosed by the absence of withdrawal bleeding when both estrogen and progestins are administered. A hysterosalpingogram or hysteroscopy can demonstrate intrauterine adhesions in many of these patients.

In those patients using no method, or one of the less reliable methods, of contraception, a serum pregnancy test should be obtained prior to the administration of each cycle of progestin, since the possibility of a spontaneous, unexpected ovulation and subsequent pregnancy could occur. Furthermore, the patient should be cautioned not to become complacent in the use of her contraceptive because of her knowledge that ovulation is occurring rarely, if at all. Spontaneous ovulations in such patients are not rare. In such a situation, the fetus could be unnecessarily exposed to progestins during its early development, increasing the risk of limb and cardiac abnormalities.[26,27] Progesterone can also be used as a progestational agent. It is administered as an intramuscular injection. There perhaps is less risk of birth defects when this naturally occurring hormone is used.[28] However, its administration requires the added expense of an office visit. It should also be remembered that the administration of progesterone can occasionally cause a spontaneous ovulation to occur,[29] delaying withdrawal bleeding for 14 days rather than the expected withdrawal within 7 days following the injection.

Other Problems

Other causes of abnormal uterine bleeding have been previously listed, and include: emotional stress, ovarian failure, pituitary tumor, hyperprolactinemia, or an abnormality of another endocrine system. These will most likely result in oligo- or amenorrhea rather than frequent episodes of irregular vaginal bleeding.

Ovulatory patients can also have abnormal uterine bleeding. One of the more common causes is the periovulatory bleeding that occurs in some women secondary to the transient midcycle decline in estrogen that occurs normally in all ovulatory women. If the amount of estrogen falls below the critical threshold level necessary for endometrial stability, spotting can occur. The diagnosis is suggested by cyclical mid-cycle bleeding in a woman with an ovulatory basal temperature curve. Reassurance is the only therapy indicated, although the symptoms will cease if the woman takes oral contraceptives to inhibit ovulation.

Pre-menstrual staining can occur in women with a decreased amount of progesterone in the latter portion of the luteal phase. This results in a partial progesterone withdrawal. The diagnosis can be made by an out-of-phase endometrial biopsy performed in the late luteal phase. Endometriosis is also associated with such symptomatology.[30]

Hypermenorrhea (or menorrhagia) can be associated with an anatomic abnormality of the uterus, coagulopathies, or seemingly no recognizable problem. In these cases, the most effective form of therapy is to treat or remove the anatomical problem, such as a submucus myoma or endometrial polyp. Oral contraceptives and certain intrauterine devices are associated with a decreased proliferation of endometrium and can be tried in certain patients. There are, however, a few patients in this group for whom hysterectomy is the only cure for the problem. This becomes necessary if menses result in repeated massive loss of red blood cell volume.

Ectopic Pregnancy, Threatened Abortion, and Pelvic Inflammatory Disease Presenting as Vaginal Bleeding

These three conditions are discussed separately since the emergency room physician has a special obligation to differentiate carefully each of them from the other, and since all three can be associated with abnormal vaginal bleeding. In particular, the possibility of ectopic gestation should always be borne in mind, for this condition has more than once been inappropriately treated with bedrest (for impending abortion), oral contraceptives (for anovulation), or intramuscular penicillin (for pelvic inflammation), with morbid or even fatal results. The availability of sensitive and rapid tests for circulating chorionic gonadotropin has markedly increased the effectiveness of such procedures for diagnosing ectopic pregnancy, despite the decreased amounts of the hormone present in this condition. Graphs are available showing the amount of human chorionic gonadotropin expected at a particular stage of a normal pregnancy. A lower than expected level should point to either impending abortion or an ectopic gestation. Particular attention should be directed to the patient who has had previous tubal surgery or who experiences abnormal bleeding accompanied by pain. It should be remembered that pain sometimes does not occur until late in the course of an ectopic gestation. Ultrasonographic examination of the pelvis can reveal an intrauterine gestational sac or confirm a suspected adnexal mass. However, regardless of the results of laboratory testing, the physician's degree of suspicion is frequently the most important variable. Culdocentesis should not be employed except in rare situations because of the misleading information that can result. If the index of suspicion for ectopic pregnancy is great enough that such a maneuver is considered, and the corroborating laboratory tests have not conclusively ruled out the possibility of an extrauterine gestation, then laparoscopy is the diagnostic tool of choice. Such early intervention is particularly important in light of the increasing use of conservative tubal surgery in young patients desiring the possibility of future childbearing.

BLEEDING IN THE OLDER PATIENT (OVER AGE 35)

There is an increasing probability that an anatomic problem is the cause of abnormal vaginal bleeding in older women, although an anatomic etiology for vaginal bleeding can occur in any age group. These anatomic abnormalities include: endocervical or endometrial polyps; cancer of the cervix, endometrium, or tube; hormonally active tumors of the ovary; uterine leiomyomas, particularly of the submucus variety; chronic endometritis including tuberculosis; chronic cervicitis; and adenomyosis or endometriosis (Table 7.4).

Although nonfunctional etiologies are more common in this age group,

Table 7-4. Causes of bleeding in the older patient.

Anatomic abnormalities—polyps, cancers, hormonally active tumors, leiomyomas, endometritis, adenomyosis, endometriosis
Endocrinologic abnormalities
Anovulatory bleeding

peri-menopausal women frequently have anovulatory, and thus irregular, bleeding episodes. Most women menstruate regularly throughout their reproductive life, and, when ovarian function ceases, menstrual periods stop abruptly without further bleeding. For others, however, the years preceding the climacteric may be highlighted with episodes of irregular bleeding which frequently may be heavy or occur often enough to produce anemia secondary to chronic blood loss. Most women who develop post-menopausal bleeding are usually fearful of the diagnosis of cancer. As a result some of these patients delay the initial visit to their physician for fear that their suspicions will be confirmed. The majority, however, seek immediate medical attention, on occasion in their local hospital's emergency room.

In this age group, tissue sampling of the endometrium is mandatory because of the increased incidence of malignancy. In 401 patients with post-menopausal bleeding, Pacheco and Kempers (1968)[31] showed that 16 percent had endometrial cancer and 1 percent had cervical cancer. The other diagnoses found were benign. Latour and Pelletier (1961)[32] found a 9.8 percent incidence of carcinoma of the endometrium and 13.3 percent incidence of carcinoma of the cervix in 2,000 post-menopausal women who had vaginal bleeding. Keirse (1973)[33] found a 23 percent incidence of malignancy in 160 cases of post-menopausal bleeding. Although most women with post-menopausal bleeding do not have a malignancy, each patient should be evaluated with a Papanicolou smear, biopsy of cervical lesions or areas not stained with Schiller's solution, bimanual examination to detect irregular uterine enlargement or adnexal masses, and some type of sampling of the uterine lining.

The time-honored method for sampling uterine tissue in the post-menopausal female has been the fractional uterine curettage. This also allows a thorough pelvic examination while the patient is anesthetized. It is possible to simultaneously perform a laparoscopy, hysteroscopy, or hysterosalpingogram if these would be of assistance in diagnosing problems such as fibroids (particularly the submucosal variety), polyps, or questionable adnexal masses. In the case of adnexal masses that are definitely palpated, laparotomy is the initial treatment of choice. The diagnostic strategy for these cases is based on several factors, including the class of the pap smear, the normality of the pelvic examination, the general health of the patient, and the previous history of abnormal bleeding. Several physicians advocate one of the various in-office procedures to sample the endometrial cavity. These include techniques for histological sampling, such as the use of an endometrial biopsy instrument or the Vabra suction aspirator. The Gravlee jet wash provides a sample for cytological evaluation. All of these instruments can be used without the added cost of a hospitalization. Moreover, it has been reported that the endometrial cavity can be sounded in more than 90 percent of women with post-menopausal bleeding,[34] hence such in-office procedures are potentially feasible in the majority of post-menopausal women. Patient discomfort, although real with these procedures, is thought to be minimized by gentleness and a careful explanation. Marshall (1974)[35] reports that no endometrial carcinomas have gone undetected with the use of a thorough in-office curettage. The accuracy of the Gravlee jet washer is reported at 93 to 94 percent,[36] and of the Vabra aspirator at 83 to 92 percent.[34] Nevertheless, many physicians find that women must be carefully selected for such diagnostic maneuvers, chiefly because of the degree of discomfort involved. When an in-office procedure does not seem appropriate, a cervical dilation and uterine curettage can be performed utilizing an intravenous analgesic and a paracervical block. General anesthesia should, however, be immediately available if it is needed. A hospital stay for only a few hours is usually sufficient to identify any complications if they occur.

Even in post-menopausal patients, the histopathology following uterine sampling is most frequently benign. Atrophic endometrium may represent endometrium stimulated by low amounts of estrogen sufficient to cause bleeding but not proliferation; it may also represent an exhausted endometrium following a prolonged bleeding episode. About half of the endometrial biopsies performed for post-menopausal bleeding are taken from patients being treated with estrogens,[35] and the greater the dosage of estrogen, the more likely will endometrial sampling for bleeding be necessary.[35] Locally-administered estrogen preparations are rapidly absorbed and can also produce abnormal bleeding.[37] Extraglandular production of increased amounts of estrone from circulating androstenedione can occur in post-menopausal women not taking exogenous estrogen. This results from an increased production of androstenedione or an increased peripheral conversion of androstenedione to estrone in patients with obesity, liver disease, or virilizing ovarian tumors. Women with obesity, hypertension, diabetes, or infertility appear more prone to develop endometrial malignancy over and above any other consideration.[38]

Exogenous estrogens increase the risk of endometrial cancer about 4.5 times when compared to women not exposed to such estrogen therapy.[39] Luteal phase progesterone in the ovulatory woman produces a reduction in estradiol receptors and an increased metabolism of estradiol to the weaker estrogen, estrone.[40] Because of these findings, Gambrell (1977)[34] has suggested that progestins be given to all women undergoing post-menopausal estrogen replacement. He contends that the cyclical bleeding that may follow progestin administration is controlled and avoids overproliferation of the endometrium that can occur when estrogens are given alone. In his experience, progestins not only produce a more complete sloughing of the endometrium, but also convert hyperplastic endometrial changes to secretory endometrium in nearly all cases. Gambrell and Greenblatt (1975)[41] have shown that even severe atypical adenomatous hyperplasia reverts to normal after three cycles of norgestrel 0.5 mg and ethinyl estradiol 0.05 mg (Ovral). The medication is given initially 3 times a day for 1 day. This is followed by 1 tablet twice a day for the next 9 days. After a 7-day drug-free interval, 1 tablet is taken daily for 21 additional days over the next 2 subsequent cycles. With this therapy, hyperplastic endometrium, regardless of its degree of atypicality, has almost invariably been found to revert to normal. Acute heavy bleeding can be arrested in 6 to 48 hours when this regimen is employed.[41] When bleeding is slight, or has ceased, 5 mg of norethindrone acetate (Norlutate) is administered for 7 days each month, usually from the 19th to the 25th day of the month. Patients with hyperplasia of the endometrium who are so treated must have a repeat office curettage after 3 months of therapy to verify that hyperplastic changes no longer persist. If hyperplasia is again found, a hysterectomy should be performed. Once progestin therapy is initiated in a post-menopausal woman, it is continued until the patient has 3 months without withdrawal uterine bleeding. Withdrawal bleeding begins from 2 to 7 days after the last progestin tablet is taken and rarely lasts longer than 3 to 5 days. Any variation from this pattern requires a repeat office curettage. Patients presenting with post-menopausal bleeding while undergoing estrogen replacement therapy are continued on the estrogen, and progestin is added after a diagnostic uterine sampling is performed. Women on cyclic estrogens, such as from the first to the 25th day of the month, who have bleeding occurring only at the end of the month (estrogen-withdrawal bleeding) are not subjected to a uterine sampling procedure. Instead, a progestin is added for the last 7 days of each month's estrogen course. If breakthrough or irregular bleeding occurs, a complete evaluation is performed, including a sampling of the endometrium.

Therapy in each woman should be individualized. For instance, an older, pre-menopausal woman with persistent bleeding might be optimally treated with a hysterectomy if her family has been completed, and a pre-operative endometrial sampling has not identified a malignancy.

TREATMENT OF UNRESPONSIVE VAGINAL BLEEDING

Occasionally very heavy vaginal hemorrhage is unresponsive to hormonal or simple surgical (curettage) therapies. In these cases, hysterectomy or hypogastric artery ligation or embolization is necessary to achieve hemostasis. It should be remembered that true vaginal bleeding, i.e., bleeding not originating from the uterus, will not be controlled by ligation of the hypogastric arterial system. Nevertheless, such measures are applicable not only for intractable uterine hemorrhage, but also can be used in cases of massive pelvic trauma and complications of a pregnancy.

Baumgartner,[42] reported the successful control of hemorrhage from a human carcinoma in 1888 by ligation of both hypogastric arteries. Miller (1963)[43] published the first article describing the successful use of hypogastric artery ligation in cases of massive pelvic injuries secondary to traumatic crush injuries of the bony pelvis. Although there has been reported control of uterine bleeding by the selective installation of vasoconstrictor agents such as vasopressin,[44] in general, vasoconstrictor therapy has not been successful in pelvic bleeding secondary to trauma.[45] Attention has thus been directed to transcatheter embolization of particulate matter to achieve hemostasis within the pelvis. Ligation of the hypogastric arteries in such situations occasionally proves technically difficult or impossible and has the disadvantage of releasing the tamponading effect of the contained pelvic hematoma. Transcatheter embolization of the hypogastric arteries circumvents this problem and has proven very effective in some situations.[45] Gelfoam and autogenous blood clots have been successfully utilized. Balloon catheters in the hypogastric arteries have also been effective in controlling hemorrhage secondary to crush injuries of the pelvis. Nonetheless, the mainstay for control of massive pelvic hemorrhage is surgical extirpation of the affected organ. These alternate therapies, although proven effective in certain situations, should be employed only in medical centers which have experience in their use.

REFERENCES

1. Novak ER, Jones GS, Jones Jr, HW: Novak's Textbook of Gynecology. Williams and Wilkins, Baltimore, 1970.
2. Heller ME, Savage MO, Dewhurst J: Vaginal bleeding in childhood: a review of 51 patients. Br J Obstet Gynaecol 85:721–725, 1978.
3. Wilkins L: The Diagnosis and Treatment of Endocrine Disorders in Childhood and Adolescence. Charles C. Thomas, Springfield IL, 1965.
4. Pedowitz P, Felmus LB, Mackles A: Precocious pseudopuberty due to ovarian tumors. Obstet Gynecol Surv 10:633–653, 1955.
5. Herbst AL, Kurman RJ, Scully RE, Poskanzer DC: Clear-cell adenocarcinoma of the genital tract in young females. N Engl J Med 287:1259–1264, 1972.
6. Smith RF, Dunkelberg Jr WE: Inhibition of Corynebacterium vaginale by metronidazole. Sex Transm Dis 4:20–21, 1977.
7. Huffman JW: Premenarchal vulvovaginitis. Clin Obstet Gynecol 20:581–593, 1977.
8. Brenner PF: Precocious puberty in the female. In Mishell Jr, DR, Davajan V, Eds: Reproductive Endocrinology, Infertility and Contraception. F.A. Davis, Philadelphia, 1979.
9. Altchek A: Dysfunctional uterine bleeding in adolescence. Clin Obstet Gynecol 20:633–650, 1977.
10. March CM: Luteal phase defects. In Mishell Jr, DR, Davajan V, Eds: Reproductive Endocrinology, Infertility and Contraception. F.A. Davis, Philadelphia, 1979.
11. Mishell Jr DR: Early gestation. In Mishell Jr, DR, Davajan V, Eds: Reproductive Endocrinology, Infertility and Contraception. F.A. Davis, Philadelphia, 1979.
12. Brenner PF: Androgen excess. In Mishell Jr, DR, Davajan V, Eds: Reproductive Endocrinology, Infertility and Contraception. F.A. Davis, Philadelphia, 1979.
13. Seppala M: Prolactin and female reproduction. Ann Clin Res 10:164–170, 1978.
14. Chamlian DL, Taylor HB: Endometrial hyperplasia in young women. Obstet Gynecol, 36:659–666, 1970.
15. Wiqvist N, Widholm O, Nillius SJ, Nilsson B, Eds: Dysmenorrhea and prostaglandins. Acta Obstet Gynecol Scand (Suppl) 87:1–117, 1979.
16. Givens JR: Polycystic ovarian disease. In Givens JR, Ed: Gynecologic Endocrinology. Year Book Medical Publishers, Chicago, 1977.
17. Givens JR: Hirsutism and hyperandrogenism. In Stollerman GH, Ed: Advances in Internal Medicine. 21. Year Book Medical Publishers, Chicago, 1976.

18. Abraham GE, Maroulis GB, Boyers SP, Buster JE, Magyar DM, Elsner CW: Dexamethasone suppression test in the management of hyperandrogenized patients. Obstet Gynecol, 57:158–165, 1981.
19. Abraham GE, Maroulis GB, Buster JE, et al: Effect of dexamethazone on serum cortisol and androgen levels in hirsute patients. Obstet Gynecol 47:395–402, 1976.
20. Strickler RC, Warren JC: Hirsutism: diagnosis and management. In Pitkin RM, Zlatnik FJ, Eds: 1979 Year Book of Obstetrics and Gynecology. Year Book Medical Publishers, Chicago, 1979.
21. Osborn RH, Yannone ME: Plasma androgens in the normal and androgenic female. Obstet Gynecol Surv 26:195–228, 1971.
22. Speroff L, Glass RH, Kase NG: Clinical Gynecologic Endocrinology and Infertility. Williams and Wilkins, Baltimore, 1978.
23. Yen SSC: Chronic anovulation. In Yen SSC, Jaffe RB, Eds: Reproductive Endocrinology. W.B. Saunders, Philadelphia, 1978.
24. Givens JR, Andersen RN, Wiser WL, et al: The effectiveness of two oral contraceptives in suppressing plasma androstenedione, testosterone, LH, and FSH, and in stimulating plasma testosterone-binding capacity in hirsute women. Am J Obstet Gynecol 124:333–339, 1976.
25. Kirschner MA, Jacobs JB: Combined ovarian and adrenal vein catheterization to determine the site(s) of androgen overproduction in hirsute women. J Clin Endocrinol Metab 33:199–209, 1971.
26. Janerich DT, Piper JM, Glebatis DM: Oral contraceptives and congenital limb-reduction defects. N Engl J Med 291:697–700, 1974.
27. Heinonen OP, Slone D, Monson RR, et al: Cardiovascular birth defects and antenatal exposure to female sex hormones. N Engl J Med 296:67–70, 1977.
28. Chez RA: Proceedings of the symposium "Progesterone, progestins and fetal development." Fertil Steril 30:16–26, 1978.
29. Goldenberg RL, Grodin JM, Vaitukaitis JL, Ross GT: Withdrawal bleeding and luteinizing hormone secretion following progesterone in women with amenorrhea. Am J Obstet Gynecol 115:193–196, 1973.
30. Wentz AC: Premenstrual spotting: its association with endometriosis but not luteal phase inadequacy. Fertil Steril 33:605–607, 1980.
31. Pacheco JC, Kempers RD: Etiology of postmenopausal bleeding. Obstet Gynecol 32:40–46, 1968.
32. Latour JPA, Pelletier JP: Incidence of uterine malignancy in postmenopausal bleeders. Am J Obstet Gynecol 81:146–147, 1961.
33. Keirse MJ: Aetiology of postmenopausal bleeding. Postgrad Med J 49:344–348, 1973.
34. Gambrell Jr RD: Postmenopausal bleeding. Clin Obstet Gynaecol 4:129–143, 1977.
35. Marshall BR: Postmenopausal vaginal bleeding during estrogen therapy. JAMA 227:76–77, 1974.
36. Kistner RW, Krantz KE, Lebherz TB, et al: Endometrial cancer: rising incidence, detection and treatment. J Reprod Med 10:53–74, 1973.
37. Schiff I, Tulchinsky D, Ryan KJ: Vaginal absorption of estrone and 17B estradiol. Fertil Steril 28:1063–1066, 1977.
38. Mickal A, Torres J: Adenocarcinoma of the endometrium. In Greenblatt RB, Mahesh VB, McDonough PG, Eds: The Menopausal Syndrome. Medcom Press, New York, 1974.
39. Smith DC, Prentice R, Thompson DJ, Herrman WL: Association of exogenous estrogen and endometrial carcinoma. N Engl J Med 293, 1164–1167, 1975.

40. Gurpide E, Tseng L: Factors controlling intracellular levels of estrogens in human endometrium. Gynecol Oncol 2:221–227, 1974.
41. Gambrell Jr RD, Greenblatt RB: Management of dysfunctional uterine bleeding with norgestrel-ethinyl estradiol. Current Med Dialog 42:80–85, 1975.
42. Leventhal ML, Lash AF, Grossman A: Hemorrhage from carcinoma of the cervix: control by extraperitoneal ligation of the hypogastric arteries. Surg Gynecol Obstet 67:102–105, 1938.
43. Miller WE: Massive hemorrhage in fractures of the pelvis. South Med J 56:933–938, 1963.
44. Pavlin V, Flynn MJ, Mulder JL, Cort JH: The treatment of uterine bleeding with vasopressin hormonogen (glypressin)—a pilot study. Br J Obstet Gynecol 85:801–805, 1978.
45. Smith DC, Wyatt JF: Embolization of hypogastric arteries in the control of massive vaginal hemorrhage. Obstet Gynecol 49:317–322, 1977.

8 Contraceptive Problems

Jan Schneider

The choice of a contraceptive method for any woman must take into account both its effectiveness and its risk. It is a harsh truth that the methods which most reliably prevent pregnancy also carry the greatest incidence of health complications. Many such complications are of a nature which may cause the patient to present to the emergency room.

When any patient is initially counseled about choice of family planning method, the effectiveness and risk must be carefully explained to her. In most healthy women the ultimate choice will be a very personal one, based upon individual perception of the need for protection against pregnancy balanced against concerns about risks and side effects.

The effectiveness of a method of contraception is measured by its incidence of failure, the pregnancy rate. This is derived by the so-called Pearl formula as the number of pregnancies per 100 woman-years of exposure. The theoretical model is the woman at risk of pregnancy for 100 years or, in more realistic terms, the number of pregnancies per 100 women using the method in any given year. This can be stated as a percentage risk. If no method of contraception is used the pregnancy rate is in the range of 65 to 85. Any method of contraception which can bring the pregnancy rate down to 10 or less is considered effective enough to be acceptable. The most effective contraceptives ever devised are the oral estrogen-progesterone agents together referred to as the "PILL." Oral estrogen-progestin agents bring the pregnancy rate down to one or less. There is no other drug in the pharmacopeia which is as effective in doing that which it was designed to do as is the oral contraceptive in avoiding pregnancy. More than a third of contraceptive users in the United States have elected this method and currently there are between 7 and 12 million women taking oral contraceptives in this country.[1]

Second in effectiveness is the intrauterine contraceptive device. Use of an IUD brings the pregnancy rate down to between 2 and 4; those containing metallic copper or impregnated with progesterone are somewhat more effective than those of plastic alone. About 10 percent of contraceptive users in the United States wear an IUD. Third in effectiveness are the various methods based upon chemical spermicidal activity. The diaphragm, which has its effect primarily by holding the spermicidal cream or jelly against the cervix, brings the pregnancy rate down to the range of 7 or 8. The effectiveness is clearly a function not only of the method itself, but of the motivation of the patient to use it and her ability to do so. The vaginal foams used alone are slightly less effective than the diaphragm and carry a pregnancy rate around 8 to 10. The foaming tablets, which do contain a spermicidal agent similar to the foam, are less effective than the foam because it may take time for the tablet to melt in the vagina and the agent may not be spread evenly. Finally, the barrier method that uses the condom has a pregnancy rate around 8 to 10. This also is determined by motivation but can be significantly enhanced if used together with a vaginal foam.

For the physician working in an emergency room, the diaphragm, spermicidal agents, and condoms rarely pose much of a problem. Occasionally a patient has difficulty removing a diaphragm or forgets that one is left in place and this may be a surprise finding on pelvic exam. Once in a while sensitivity to one or other of the spermicidal agents may cause vaginal, vulvar, or penile irritation and rash. This is most easily treated by discontinuation of use. Occasionally topical steroids must be used. A condom may slip from the penis to become a vaginal foreign body and be discovered as a cause of discharge. However, these most simple but least effective methods are unlikely to pose much of a health concern other than the problems of pregnancy due to failure.

ORAL CONTRACEPTIVES

When considering the complications of oral contraception both minor side effects and major complications must be considered (Table 8.1). The minor side effects became much publicized when the oral contraceptives were first marketed. These were mainly of nuisance value and have remarkably diminished in

Table 8-1. Complications of oral contraceptives.

Complications
Minor Complications
Nausea
Weight gain
Fluid retention
Mastalgia
Breakthrough bleeding
Amenorrhea
Major Complications
Thromboembolic disease
Intracranial vascular catastrophes
Hypertension
Hepatocellular adenoma
Post-pill amenorrhea

severity and frequency as the dose of both estrogenic and progesterone components has been reduced.

Minor Complications

Nausea was a common side effect presumably related to the estrogen level. Many patients complained of weight gain and fluid retention; these were ascribed to the progesterone component and were probably caused by the anabolic effects of the testosterone-like composition of the synthetic progestins. Many patients also complained of some mastalgia; this was also due to the progestin component. One minor problem which has continued in spite of the low dosage of the modern agents is breakthrough bleeding. The low levels of estrogen and progesterone may not stimulate the endometrium enough to maintain it fully for the full 28 days, and some mid-cycle spotting is not uncommon. The low level of hormones may cause the endometrium to be stimulated so little that at the end of 21 days of pill ingestion, no bleeding will occur. Occasionally 2 or 3 months of amenorrhea will occur; this may cause concern and confusion about the possibility of pregnancy. The low level of contraceptive failure if the pills have been taken regularly almost mitigates against this possibility; nonetheless, evaluation of the patient is indicated. Another complication, which was not uncommon with higher level of estrogen and progesterone, is that of sloughing of a complete cast of the endometrium. In patients *not* on oral contraception this sign remains an ominous indication of possible ectopic pregnancy.

Major Complications

Thromboembolic and Intracranial Disease. For everything there is a price, and the major systemic health complications of oral contraception have been highly publicized. The most serious of these are the thromboembolic diseases and intracranial vascular catastrophes. Patients taking oral estrogen-progestins have a risk of venous thrombosis and embolization 3 to 5 times greater than do women who do not take oral contraception.[2,3,4,5] The risk was greater when higher levels of estrogen were used, although the exact dose relationship to risk has not been established. The newer medications, with less than 50 micrograms of the estrogen, are widely believed to have a much smaller risk than did the original agents, yet most available data are from a time when the higher dose was commonly used. An estimate of one case per thousand women per year is a fair assessment of the risk. The incidence of thromboembolism increases with age and it is widely agreed that this method of contraception should not be used over the age of 35. The risk, however, does not seem to be related to the duration of use of the medication. The risk of thromboembolization is particularly increased in patients who have had surgery, particularly abdominal or pelvic surgery, or who are compelled to sustain prolonged immobilization. Under such situations it is wise to discontinue oral contraception if possible.

Intracranial catastrophe in patients using oral contraception is more likely to be due to thrombotic rather than to hemorrhagic disease; however, hypertension due to these agents may cause the latter. Various studies in England and the United States have noted the risk of intracranial catastrophe to increase from 4 to 9 fold in users of oral contraceptives.[3,4,5] It has been calculated that approximately 1 in every 4000 users will have such a diagnosis for each year of use.[6] This risk, although very small, is one which patients must be warned about.

Hypertension. A second serious medical complication associated with oral contraceptives is hypertension. A significant elevation of blood pressure is noted in up to 19 percent of oral contraceptive users. The incidence clearly is affected by the criteria used to diagnose hypertension.[7,8] More than half of women who develop hypertension for the first time while on oral contraceptives revert back to a normal blood pressure once the medication is discontinued. The importance of checking blood pressure at each return visit is obvious and is probably more important than is the usual routine pelvic exam.

Hepatocellular Adenoma. Hepatocellular adenoma has recently been described as having a significantly increased incidence in patients on oral contraceptives. The occurrence of this rare tumor of the liver is also directly associated with the duration of oral contraceptive use.[9,10] After 6 to 8 years of oral contraceptive use, the incidence of hepatocellular adenoma is 18 times greater than in patients who do not use the medication. Fifty percent of women with hepatocellular adenoma have been on oral contraceptives for more than 5 years. The tumor is very vascular and may cause massive intraabdominal hemorrhage. The mortality of its complications may be as high as 8 percent. The usual presenting symptom is severe abdominal or thoracic pain, frequently of sudden onset. Other patients have recurrent episodes of minor pain, sometimes associated with syncope. In approximately 40 percent of patients, the first symptom is the finding of an abdominal mass. Frequently this mass is found by the patient herself. There has been some suggestion that symptoms are most common at the time of menses, although this has not been confirmed.

Post-pill Amenorrhea. Although there is no long-term impact on fertility in patients who use oral contraception, the incidence of post-pill amenorrhea with or without galactorrhea has been clearly established. Between 0.2 and 0.8 percent of patients who have been on oral contraception for some time experience delay before the re-establishment of their spontaneous menstrual function.[11,12] The incidence is probably most marked in patients who have had oligomenorrhea prior to starting oral contraception, or who have never adequately established an ovular menstrual pattern. Patients with a suggestive history should not be given oral contraceptives until the presence of normal ovular function has been demonstrated.

Usually post-pill amenorrhea is self-limited, with spontaneous resumption of normal cycles. The only emergency problem related to this may be that of evaluating gestational age by history in patients who become pregnant prior to the onset of what would have been the first menstrual period.

Coronary Disease and Cancer. Coronary disease, although rare in women, does increase with age, and has a clear association with smoking. However, there have been several studies which indicate that there is *no* increased risk of myocardial infarction which can be ascribed to the use of oral contraception. Furthermore, there has been *no* demonstrated correlation between malignancy of the genital tract and oral contraception; malignancy of the cervix, endometrium, ovary, or breast is not increased in women who are or have been on oral contraceptives.

The complications of oral contraception cannot be denied. A few may present as acute emergencies. A diagnosis of thromboembolic disease, intracranial catastrophe, hypertension, abdominal pain, or upper abdominal mass in any woman merits a full contraceptive history.

INTRAUTERINE CONTRACEPTIVE DEVICES

The intrauterine contraceptive devices, once inserted, have the advantage of requiring no act of memory or planning by either sexual partner. However, they do carry certain risks and complications; these have been subject to considerable adverse publicity. It must be noted, however, that the United States Food and Drug Administration has declared: "IUCD's are a generally safe, effective and useful form of birth control." Complications associated with use of this method of contraceptive are discussed below (Table 8.2).

Expulsion

Between 5 and 20 percent of patients have spontaneous expulsion of the intrauterine contraceptive device within a year of insertion. The incidence of expulsion is greater in patients who have never been pregnant. It would appear that the uterus accepts the foreign body better after a pregnancy; yet there is also an age factor, since older patients retain their IUD better than the young, irrespective of parity. The highest incidence of spontaneous expulsion occurs when the IUD is inserted soon after a pregnancy, whether it terminated by abortion or delivery. If the device itself is not seen, the usual first evidence that it has been expelled is the patient noticing that the string (or strings, depending on the model) can no longer be palpated. Not infrequently the expelled IUD remains in the vagina until the time of a bowel movement, when it may be

Table 8-2. Complications of IUD's.

Expulsion
Perforation
Bleeding
Intrauterine pregnancy
Ectopic pregnancy
Infection

expressed without being noticed. When a patient presents with the complaint of the IUD strings no longer being palpated, there are three possibilities: the strings may have been drawn up into the uterus, the device may have been expelled, or perforation may have occurred.

Perforation

The risk of an IUD perforating the fundus or cervix of the uterus is probably greatest at the time of insertion. Occasionally the uterine sound or the introducer may be recognized as having perforated the uterus, frequently with minimal discomfort to the patient. At other times nothing is noted at the time of insertion. Only when the strings can no longer be palpated is it realized that the IUD is lost. Occasionally perforation of the uterus by the IUD occurs much later than the time of introduction; however, it must be assumed that at least the initiation of the perforation may have occurred at the time the IUD was inserted. Therefore the risk of perforation must be considered to be increased in those models of intrauterine contraceptive device which require frequent change and reinsertion. The overall perforation rate has been reported in various series to be between 1 and 8 per thousand introductions: 2 per thousand is frequently considered to represent a priori risk.[13]

A patient who presents with a lost IUD must be assessed as to whether it remains in the uterus, has perforated, or has been expelled. A pelvic examination is essential. Occasionally the string can be seen, although the patient was unable to palpate it. If the string cannot be seen, the uterus may be probed; once in a while the tip of the device can be discerned or may even be pulled down with a hook. When all this fails, radiologic studies should be ordered. Since all IUD's currently used are impregnated with barium, they are radiopaque and can be seen on an X-ray plate. Though an X-ray will establish that a device is present, it may not be able to identify where. The second step, therefore, is to discover whether the IUD is in or out of the uterus. The easiest method of doing this is to insert a metal sound into the uterus and take AP and lateral X-rays to assess whether the sound is in contact with the IUD. Another method is to introduce a second IUD and judge the distance between the two. If the distance is so great that it is evident that both cannot be in the uterus, perforation into the abdominal cavity must be presumed. Ultrasonography has also been used to locate a lost intrauterine device. Ultrasound has the advantage of depth perception, so a second object need not be introduced. However, the accuracy of diagnosis depends upon the skill of the ultrasonographer. Lippes Loop IUD's are more easily noted on ultrasound than the simpler shape of a Copper 7 or Copper T.

When perforation of the uterus occurs, most authorities agree that the device should be removed from the peritoneal cavity. Closed ring devices such as the Birnberg Bow (which is rarely used today) carry the risk of intestinal strangulation, should the bowel work its way into the ring. This risk does not occur with such open devices as the Lippes Loop, 7, or T. Although these are not likely to cause strangulation, the risks of infection, formation of adhesions, and even perforation of the bowel have been described: therefore, most agree that whenever perforation of the uterus by an IUD occurs, the device should be removed.[14,15] This can be achieved most simply by laparoscopy.

Bleeding

A series of bleeding problems may occur with the device. Most women note that their periods are both heavy and prolonged when an IUD is worn. Studies have shown that the amount of blood lost with each menstrual period is approximately doubled. Intermenstrual spotting is also common, occurring most frequently soon after introduction. When a device has remained in utero for several years, a deposition of calcific salts causes the once smooth plastic to be roughened and saw-like; the result may be a mechanical erosion of the endometrium and spotting. Bleeding complications are the most frequent cause for medically indicated removal of an IUD. From 12 to 16 percent of patients in various studies have the IUD removed in each year of use because of this or some other medical indication.[13]

Pregnancy

Intrauterine pregnancy occurs in about 2 to 4 percent of IUD users each year. Such pregnancies may co-exist with an IUD; however, there is a significant risk of spontaneous abortion when this happens. The incidence of abortion may be as high as 50 percent. This is particularly dangerous because abortion in the presence of a foreign body is associated with a significant incidence of sepsis. It is because of this risk that an IUD should be removed immediately when a pregnancy is diagnosed, unless the strings have been drawn up into the uterus. The removal of the IUD may itself precipitate a spontaneous abortion but the risk of this occurring is less than the 50 percent which would occur if the IUD were left and it does obviate the hazard of sepsis even if the pregnancy were lost.

Ectopic Pregnancy

The relative incidence of ectopic pregnancy in the presence of an IUD is significantly increased. There continues to be argument whether the incidence of ectopic pregnancy is increased absolutely as well as relatively. The IUD has its contraceptive effect by preventing intrauterine pregnancy, but may be assumed to have no influence upon the incidence of ectopic pregnancy. The relative increase of ectopics can therefore be easily explained. Because the incidence of ectopic pregnancy seems to be greater in IUD wearers than would be expected, many believe the increased incidence to be absolute as well as relative. Approximately 5 percent of all pregnancies in IUD wearers are ectopic. Patients with an IUD who present with pain, bleeding, or any of the other symptoms of an ectopic pregnancy must be evaluated with particular care.

Infection

The presence of a foreign body in the uterus may cause infection, even in the absence of spontaneous incomplete abortion.[16,17] The incidence of infection seems to be particularly high in nulligravidas, whose uteri, as stated above, seem to be less receptive to the presence of a foreign body in every way. Upper genital tract infection is 4 times more common in IUD wearers than in the total population; in nulligravidas, the relative risk is increased 7 fold. The greatest increase is of nongonorrheal salpingitis. When infection occurs, the device should be removed, but high-dose antibiotics should be given before removal, to reduce the risk of bacteremia when the device is manipulated. Infection may progress to chronic changes and abscess formation. Unilateral tubo-ovarian abscess, most unusual as a sequel of chronic gonococcal salpingitis, is particularly characteristic of chronic infection secondary to the use of an IUD. Such patients can be very ill and it is imperative that they be accurately diagnosed and aggressively treated. Ruptured tubo-ovarian abscess is a surgical emergency and demands immediate laparotomy and drainage. Pelvic actinomycosis has also been described with prolonged IUD use: occasionally actinomycosis may be noted on the cytology smear.

Cervical Changes

At one time it was postulated that there might be an increased incidence of carcinoma of the cervix due to the chronic irritation of the intrauterine string or plastic tail of some of the earlier devices; however, this has never been substantiated. Malignancy may be ruled out as a complication of the IUD. However, certain characteristic changes of cervical cytology have been described, perhaps related to the foreign body effect of the strings in the endocervix. It is important therefore to make notation of the presence of an IUD when a Papanicolaou smear is sent to the cytology laboratory.

The IUD has had a tumultuous history of repeated acceptance and rejection since the years of the Graafenberg ring. Although it holds a limited place in the United States, in other parts of the world it has become a mainstay of birth control. Its benefits are evident but its risks cannot be dismissed. The morbidity associated with the method is described above. Beyond that, there is a recognized mortality of 1 to 10 deaths per million women-years of use. This must be taken into account when the relative value of the method is assessed. Major complications with IUD use are probably less than those associated with the estrogen-progestin oral contraceptives; yet, they are serious when they do occur. Indeed, of all the methods of contraception complications of the IUD are the most likely to present as acute emergencies in the emergency room.

CONCLUSIONS

It is clear that the more effective the method of contraception, the greater are the potential medical hazards associated with its use. These must be anticipated at at time of initial counseling and must be taken into account in the patient who presents with problems in the emergency room. Although complications of contraception exact their penalty, these must be balanced against those stemming from an unwanted pregnancy. When complications occur, these must be recognized and appropriately dealt with. There is no single best method of contraception. For each patient the most appropriate method must be individually determined.

REFERENCES

1. Ravenholt RT, Rinehart W: Age-specific mortality trends in the United States relative to use of oral contraceptives. p 17. In Sciarra JJ, Zatuchni, GI, Speidel JJ, Eds: Risks, Benefits and Controversies in Fertility Control. Harper & Row, 1978.
2. Inman WHW, Vessey MP: Investigation of deaths from pulmonary, coronary and cerebral thrombosis & embolism in women of childbearing age. Br Med J 2:193, 1968.
3. Inman WHW, Vessey MP, Westerholm B, Engelund A: Thromboembolic disease and the steroidal content of oral contraceptives. A report to the committee on safety of drugs. Br Med J 2:203, 1970.
4. Vessey MP, Doll R: Investigation of relation between use of oral contraceptives and thromboembolic disease: a further report. Br Med J 2:651–657, 1969.
5. Royal College of General Practitioners: Oral Contraceptives and Health, Pitman Medical, London, 1974.
6. Vessey MP: Steroid contraception, venous thromboembolism and stroke: data from countries other than the United States. p 113. In Sciarra JJ, Zatuchni GI, Speidel JJ, Eds: Risks, Benefits and Controversies in Fertility Control. Harper & Row, 1978.
7. Tyson J: Oral contraceptives and elevated blood pressure. Am J Obstet Gynecol 100:875, 1968.
8. Spellacy WN, Birk SA: The effect of intrauterine devices, oral contraceptives, estrogens and progestogens on blood pressure. Am J Obstet Gynecol 112:912, 1972.
9. Christopherson WJ, Mays ET:Liver tumors and oral contraceptives. Lancet 1:1076, 1976.
10. Nissen ED, Kent DR: Liver tumors and oral contraceptives. Obstet Gynecol 46:460, 1975.
11. Petersson R, Fried H, Nillius SJ: Epidemiology of secondary amenorrhea. 1. Incidence and prevalence rate. Am J Obstet Gynecol 117:80–86, 1973.
12. Tyson JE, Andreasson B, Huth J, et al: Neuroendocrine dysfunction in galactorrhea-amenorrhea after oral contraceptive use. Obstet Gynecol 45:1–11, 1975.
13. Intrauterine Devices, Population Reports, Series B, No 3, May 1979 Population Information Program, The Johns Hopkins University.
14. Soderstrom RM: The wandering IUD—what to do? p 408. In Sciarra JJ, Zatuchni

GI, Speidel JJ, Eds: Risks, Benefits and Controversies in Fertility Control. Harper & Row, 1978.

15. Kirpatrick DH, Schneider J, Peterson EP: Large bowel perforation by intrauterine contraceptive devices. Obstet Gynecol 46:610, 1975.
16. Willson JR, Ledger WJ: Complications associated with the use of intrauterine contraceptive devices in women of middle and upper socioeconomic class. Am J Obstet Gynecol 100:649, 1968.
17. Mead PB, Beecham JB, Maeck JS: Incidence of infections associated with intrauterine contraceptive device in an isolated community. Am J Obstet Gynecol 125:79, 1976.

9 Vaginitis

Robert S. Weinstein

Vulvovaginitis is an extremely common disorder. It has been estimated that 25 percent of patients visiting a gynecologist present with complaints of vaginitis. The symptoms may be so severe that the patient seeks primary treatment in an emergency room. In general the correct diagnosis is easy to make. It is to the advantage of an emergency room physician to learn how to recognize quickly the different types of vaginitis and institute therapeutic measures. The symptoms of vaginitis are usually caused by infections of the vaginal epithelium, but may be due to atrophic changes, cervicitis, foreign body, gonococcal infection of the cervix, or rarely a malignancy of the cervix, uterus, or vagina. The normal healthy vagina during the reproductive years contains many types of bacteria, but predominantly Döderlein's bacillus (lactobacillus). This bacteria produces lactic acid and maintains the vaginal pH between 3.8 and 4.5. In general, organisms pathogenic to the vagina prefer a pH between 5 and 6. This pH is normally seen at menstruation, postpartum, and menopause. With a careful history about the vaginitis, inquiring about the color, odor, consistency, time of onset in relation to menstruation, and symptoms of burning or itching, or other predisposing factors, the astute physician may have a good idea of the cause of the infection before examining the patient. This chapter reviews the predisposing factors, diagnosis, and treatment of the common types of vulvovaginitis (Table 9.1).

CANDIDIASIS

Candidiasis is responsible for 40 percent of all vaginitis. It is also called moniliasis or yeast infection, and is caused by a "yeast-like" organism, Candida. There are nine varieties of Candida, the most common of which is C. albicans. This organism causes 67 percent of fungal vaginal infections. C.

Table 9-1. Factors important in diagnosis of vaginitis.

Discharge—color, odor, consistency
Time of onset during menstrual cycle
Symptoms—burning, itching
Predisposing factors—diabetes, antibiotics, age, pregnancy, obesity, chemotherapy
Miscellaneous factors—douching, sprays, deodorants, tampons

tropicalis causes 28 percent.[1] These organisms are indigenous to all human beings. They become pathogenic only when host environmental conditions are favorable for their growth. Different investigators have estimated that between 10 and 15 percent of all women are asymptomatic carriers of Candida.

Clinically, the symptoms usually present premenstrually. The patient usually complains of a thick, white vaginal discharge with severe vaginal pruritis, burning, or dyspareunia. Frequently, there is dysuria, which must be distinguished from a urinary tract infection. On examination, the vulva appears inflammed. The inflammation is usually limited to the vestibule, but there may be edema and excoriation of the labia minora extending onto the labia majora. Occasionally the infection may involve the perianal areas, and rarely may extend to the genitocrural folds, inner thighs, and buttocks; such widespread infection is more commonly associated with diabetes, pregnancy, or obesity. The vagina contains a white, caseous discharge, and the mucosa is typically deep red or violaceous, edematous, and tender. The pH is 4.0 to 4.7 (Table 9.2).

Premenstrually, there is an increase in vaginal glycogen, which is favorable for the growth of Candida. Diabetes mellitus has also been associated with frequent Candida infections, and is probably related to the associated glycosuria. It has been demonstrated that asymptomatic carriers of Candida albicans who have a glucose solution instilled intravaginally develop symptomatic infections which resolve spontaneously with cessation of the glucose.[2] Tight control of blood sugars with control of glycosuria can help prevent recurrent Candida infections in diabetics. The incidence of Candida infections in pregnancy is as high as 25 to 30 percent. This may be due to the associated increase in vaginal glycogen or glycosuria of pregnancy (related to a decreased renal threshold for glucose or altered carbohydrate metabolism with a decrease in glucose tolerance). The incidence and severity of Candida infections appear to increase with the duration of the gestation. Oral contraceptives have also been associated with Candida infections. The hormonal milieu is similar to that of pregnancy, and the estrogens induce glycogen deposition in the vaginal epithelial cells. There may also be an alteration of the patient's glucose tolerance test while on the pill. Rarely is it necessary to stop oral contraceptives because of recurrent Candida infections.[3] The use of broad-spectrum antibiotics is frequently followed by Candida infections, more often with tetracyclines

Table 9-2. Symptoms of candida vaginitis.

Thick white discharge
Premenstrual onset
Dysuria
Inflammed vulva and vagina

than penicillins. The infection most likely occurs in the asymptomatic carrier as a result of increased competition with the normal acid-forming vaginal bacilli allowing Candida overgrowth. It has also been observed that after oral tetracycline therapy, Candida increases 100- to 1000-fold in the intestinal flora and may serve as a source of vaginal infection and reinfection.[4] Patients with an altered immune status from cancer chemotherapy have an increased incidence in oral candidiasis (thrush), and vaginal candidiasis. It has also been suggested that "normal" patients with chronic Candida vaginitis may have an alteration in their cellular immune response to Candida antigens.[5]

The diagnosis of Candida vaginitis is usually suspected by the typical history and physical findings. It is easily confirmed by a wet smear prepared with a minute amount of vaginal discharge mixed with one drop of a 10 to 20 percent solution of potassium hydroxide, causing the red blood cells and white blood cells to lyse rapidly. The vaginal epithelial cells become translucent "ghost" cells. This allows the Candida to stand out clearly, under low and high power microscopic magnifications, as branching segmented filaments called mycelia or pseudohyphae. Conidia (budding yeast-like cells) may also be seen, but are not diagnostic of candidiasis since they are also seen with nonpathogenic fungi. On gram stain the mycelia are positively stained, but this test is not necessary for routine evaluation. Candida can also be cultured on Nickerson's or Sabouraud's media, but this is most helpful in experimental investigation and rarely used clinically.

The treatment of Candida vaginitis consists of using one of the many available specific antifungal agents. Nystatin vaginal suppositories (Mycostatin) may be used once daily for 2 weeks, and is not contraindicated during pregnancy. It is important not to interrupt the therapy during the menses. Antifungal vaginal creams include micronazole (Monistat 7) and clotrimazole (Gyne-lotrimin). These have become popular because they require one application daily for only 1 week. Newer regimens of clotrimazole using 2 tablets inserted at night for 3 nights have been reported to be as effective as the 7-day course. Persistent infections may require 2 weeks of use.[6] Gentian violet vaginal inserts (Genapax) have been used, but patients frequently complain of discoloration of undergarments. Many women with Candida vaginitis have a severe vulvitis which requires specific therapy. Although it has been suggested that corticosteroids may play a role in the development of Candida infections, there is no question that they are extremely helpful in treating the vulvar inflammation. Hydrocortisone cream 1 percent may be used locally 4 times daily, or a corticosteroid combined with nystatin and other local antibiotics (Mycolog cream) may be applied 3 times daily. When vulvar burning is the major complaint, the addition of cool compresses helps give more immediate relief. These compresses may consist of cool water, witch hazel, or 5 percent boric acid. One particularly soothing compress is made by dissolving a 5 grain tablet of potassium permanganate in 1 quart of cool water; this has the additional advantage of antifungal activity. Even when there is severe itching and vulvar pain oral antipruritics, i.e., hydroxyzine (Atarax) or diphenhydramine (Benedryl) and oral analgesics as codeine are rarely needed (Table 9.3).

Table 9-3. Candidiasis therapy.

Nystatin vaginal suppositories—1 qd × 14
Micronazole (Monistat 7)—qd × 7
Clotrimazole (Gyne-lotrimin)—qd × 7 or $\bar{\pi}$ qhs × 3

It is important to schedule a follow-up visit in 1 month's time to be certain that the Candida infection has been eradicated. Many recurrences are due to inadequate therapy. The patient stops taking the medication after a few days because of symptomatic relief or therapy is interrupted by the onset of menses. Many patients, after adequate therapy, will become asymptomatic carriers of Candida. They can be identified by inspection and repeat potassium hydroxide wet smear. They will remain asymptomatic until something increases the competition with the normal vaginal bacterial flora. Recurrent Candida infections can be difficult and frustrating to treat. In pregnancy, palliation may only be achieved, with rapid recovery postpartum. Screening for and controlling diabetes has been mentioned above. In patients who have recurrent Candida infections following oral antibiotics, it is worthwhile placing them on concomitant vaginal antifungal therapy during, and for 3 days beyond, the antibiotic use. Other patients note recurrences prior to each menstrual cycle, and may be helped by intravaginal treatment for 5 days prior to and 2 days during the menses for 3 to 6 cycles. Gastrointestinal candidiasis has been alluded to as a cause of recurrent vaginitis. Studies have shown that 75 percent of women with Candida vaginitis have Candida in their stools. Only 25 percent of women without vaginitis have intestinal Candida. An attempt can be made to reduce the gastrointestinal Candida flora with Nystatin oral tablets 500,000 U., 3 times a day for 10 days or until clinical cure is proven. Many patients have difficulty tolerating this medication because of intestinal distress. Candida has occasionally been shown to be sexually transmitted. It is present in the semen of husbands of women with Candida vaginitis. More commonly, Candida may secondarily infect an abrasion on the penis. This infection is usually easily treated with clotrimazole cream or Mycolog cream. The use of condoms during treatment may be helpful in prevention of vaginal recurrences. Cunnilingus has also been suggested as a cause of recurrent vaginal infections, since Candida is present in 30 percent of oral cavities. If this cause is suspected, the use of Nystatin oral suspension may be tried. Some bacteriocidal soaps, by eliminating the normal bacterial flora, have also been implicated in recurrent Candida vaginitis. This factor is easily remedied by changing to a bland soap. Nylon underwear and tight-fitting pants have also been held responsible for recurrent infections, presumably by preventing adequate ventilation and allowing moisture from perspiration to accumulate in the genital region, a factor which favors the growth of Candida. This factor can be eliminated by using cotton underwear and the newer types of pantyhose with cotton crotch inserts. When all else fails, long-term use of an acid buffered vaginal jelly (Aci-Jel) 2 or 3 times weekly for up to 6 months can be very helpful in eliminating symptomatic recurrences.[7] The large number of treatment methods and the multiple causes for recurrent infection hint at the magnitude of the problem and the difficulty the physician may have in dealing with patients with multiple recurrences.

TRICHOMONIASIS

Trichomoniasis is an extremely common vaginitis. In some reports, trichomonads have been identified in as many as 20 percent of all gynecologic patients, but the incidence has decreased in the last 10 years because of improved therapy. The infective agent, Trichomonas vaginalis, is a unicellular parasitic flagellated protozoan which fulfills Koch's postulates. It is 15 to 20 μ long and is propelled by four flagella. It is frequently symbiotic with other organisms, particularly micrococcus. This organism produces carbon dioxide gas bubbles so characteristic of Trichomonas infection. It is most prevalent in indigent populations and in individuals with poor hygiene.

Clinically, symptoms present with the onset of or following menses. The patient complains of a profuse, yellow-green, malodorous discharge which may produce an irritating vulvitis and dyspareunia. Pelvic examination may be painful with reddening of the introitus and labia minora. Occasionally, there is intertrigo of the inner thighs. The vaginal mucosa may be fiery red, or composed of multiple petechiae with patchy thinning of the epithelium. The cervix is usually friable with edema and inflammation of the cervical papillae, which gives a "strawberry" appearance. In 10 percent of the cases, the discharge is frothy in appearance, from gas-producing bacteria. Since no lactobacilli are present, the vaginal pH is less acidic, in the range of 5.1 to 5.4[8] (Table 9.4).

In addition to the acute Trichomonas infection described above, there are also asymptomatic and chronic forms. The patient with the asymptomatic infection, when questioned, usually gives a history of an acute infection in the past which resolved without specific therapy. The vaginal pH is acidic and lactobacilli are usually present with the few trichomonads. These patients are probably at risk for recurrent acute infections. The patient with chronic Trichomonas vaginitis does not complain of irritative symptoms, but does have an abnormal discharge, odor, and relatively alkaline vaginal pH, with normal-appearing vulvar and vaginal tissues. This chronic state may be maintained by the frequent use of acidifying or medicated vaginal douches.[1]

Trichomoniasis is a venereal disease in the sense that it is spread by sexual contact. The male sexual partner is usually asymptomatic, although recent studies have recovered Trichomonas vaginalis in 68 percent of men with "non-specific" urethritis.[9] Other reports have discovered T. vaginalis in 15 percent of all sexually active males and 60 percent of husbands of wives with T. vaginalis.[8] It has frequently been suggested that these organisms are harbored in the gastrointestinal tract, but T. hominis, found in the colon, and T. buccalis, found in the oral cavity, have never been proven to be vaginal pathogens. Occasionally T. vaginalis is found in the lower urinary tract, involving the urethra or the bladder. This is due to a secondary infestation following vaginitis. It is theoretically possible for the infection to be spread from infected towels.

Table 9-4. Symptoms of trichomoniasis.

Postmenstrual discharge
Profuse, yellow-green, malodorous discharge
Strawberry spots on cervix and vagina

Trichomonads have been identified in wet washcloths twenty-four hours after use, but infection from this source is most unlikely. Even less likely sources of infection include bath water, swimming pools, and toilet splash.

Estrogens and hypoacidity have been identified as predisposing factors for trichomoniasis. Trichomonas infections are seen more commonly in pregnancy, with spontaneous remission of symptoms postpartum. Similarly, postmenopausal women on estrogen therapy may develop acute Trichomonas infections more readily. An increase in vaginal pH creates a more favorable environment for Trichomonas vaginal infections. This occurs with the onset of menses (from the menstrual blood), and in patients with cervicitis because of the increased production of cervical mucus. Other vaginal bacterial infections associated with hypoacidity, especially Hemophilus vaginalis, may be related to Trichomonas infections.

The diagnosis of Trichomonas vaginitis is usually suspected from the typical history and physical findings. It can be confirmed easily with a simple technique utilizing readily available equipment. A wet smear is prepared by adding a minute amount of fresh vaginal discharge obtained from the speculum, to 1 drop of physiologic saline solution at room temperature. Trichomonads can easily be identified under low power (100 X) of a light microscope as highly motile, ovoid organisms, slightly longer than the numerous surrounding white blood cells, but one-half the size of the vaginal epithelial cells. Under high dry power (400 X), the flagella can be seen. It is important that the slide be viewed when warm, since the trichomonads become round, non-motile "pseudocysts" when allowed to cool near an open window or when suspended in cold saline. Saline solutions with bacteriostatic agents (benzyl alcohol, etc.) and water, which is not isotonic, will also impede making the diagnosis. Trichomonas vaginalis can be cultured and identified by Giemsa stain and Papanicolaou stain, but these methods are rarely required.

The successful treatment of Trichomonas vaginalis vaginitis was greatly improved in 1960 with the advent of metronidazole (Flagyl), a systemic medicine. Previous local therapies were frequently ineffective because of their inability to reach organisms located in the urinary tract or to treat male carriers. The present recommendation for metronidazole therapy is 250 mg 3 times a day for 7 days, affording a cure rate approaching 100 percent. A new regimen, becoming very popular because of the high rate of compliance, is a single dose of 2 grams (8 tablets). This has a 98 percent efficacy.[10] Since the majority of men with infected sexual partners also have asymptomatic trichomonads, it is probably best to treat them concomitantly with the same dosage schedule. Approximately one-third of the women become reinfected when the men have not been treated. Although some investigators believe that treatment of the male should be limited to reinfections or demonstration of infection in the male genital tract, this is frequently difficult from a logistic point of view. Side effects of metronidazole are minimal. They include nausea, a metallic taste, and diarrhea. In addition, patients should be warned about the use of alcohol during treatment because of a disulfiram (Antabuse)-like activity. More serious but rare side effects include bone marrow suppression, and because of this it should not be used in patients with known blood dyscrasia. Metronidazole has been proven to be carcinogenic in rodents and is contraindicated in pregnancy. Although all topical therapies have had limited success, they must still be used in patients unable to tolerate oral metronidazole, or in whom its use is contraindicated. Vaginal reacidification has been a mainstay of therapy, since trichomonads are unable to survive in a pH of less than 5. Daily use of mild acid douches for possibly as long as 30 days may be effective in 20 percent of cases. Two tablespoons of white vinegar (acetic acid) or 2 teaspoons of lactic acid per quart of warm water are used as a douching solution. Acid buffered vaginal jellies (Aci-Jel) used daily for 3 weeks have a similar effect and may be especially helpful during pregnancy in controlling symptoms until metronidazole can be used postpartum. Trichomonacidal medicated douches—polyoxyethylene monyl phenol (Vagisec)—or suppositories—furazolidone (Trichofuran)—usually need to be continued for 30 days or more, once or twice daily, and are usually ineffective in eradicating organisms in Skene's ducts or the urinary tract. The associated vulvitis can be helped with the use of a bland soap and a corticosteroid cream, such as hydrocortisone 1 percent, applied locally 4 times daily.

There are a few patients who develop recurrent infections, even after repeat metronidazole treatment of themselves and their sexual partners. Some of these women become reinfected from relations with other partners, but some may harbor trichomonads in a chronically inflammed cervix. These patients benefit from cervical cautery or cryosurgery followed by retreatment with metronidazole.

NON-SPECIFIC BACTERIAL VAGINITIS

Women presenting with a vaginal discharge who are found not to have gonorrhea, trichomoniasis, or candidiasis probably have a so-called non-specific infection. Such infections have largely gone untreated in the past and have become an ever-increasing problem. Ninety percent of these infections are due to Haemophilus vaginalis (Corynebacterium vaginale), a pleomorphic, non-motile gram-negative bacillus which is neither a true Haemophilus species nor a true Corynebacterium. It is a facultative aerobe, first described in 1953 and found only in the vagina and urethra.[11] It has been identified by various investigators in 5 to 25 percent of sexually active women. Only 50 percent of these women had a symptomatic vaginitis, but half of the asymptomatic women were found to have an offensive odor on examination.[12] The other 10 percent of non-specific bacterial vaginitis is caused by other bacteria—predominantly streptococcus, staphylococcus, and E. coli.

Patients with H. vaginalis vaginitis complain of a mild leukorrhea with a fishy offensive odor, often starting at the onset of menses or associated with urination or intercourse. There are rarely problems with significant vaginal itching, burning, or dyspareunia. Pelvic examination reveals minimal inflammation of the vulva or vagina. There is a thin gray-white vaginal discharge with the consistency of flour paste, which is frothy only 10 percent of the time. The vaginal pH is 5.0 to 5.5

Haemophilus vaginalis is probably spread by intercourse. One study identified H. vaginalis in urethral cultures of 90 percent of husbands of infected wives, but only 2.5 percent of "alleged virginal" medical students.[13] This infection in males is asymptomatic, and a study of male non-specific urethritis implicated H. vaginalis in only 1 percent of the cases. H. vaginalis prefers a less acidic pH, which is provided by a recent menstrual period. There is a high association of H. vaginalis with Trichomonas vaginalis (25 percent); this may reflect their similar pH preference as well as their venereal transmission.[14] Pessaries, retained tampons, and other foreign bodies in the vagina are predisposing factors for non-specific vaginitis. Occasionally non-specific vaginitis is associated with a profuse cervicitis, with production of copious non-acidic secretions.

The diagnosis of non-specific vaginitis is also within easy reach of the examining physician. It is partly a diagnosis of exclusion, by ruling out Trichomonas, Candida, and gonococcal infections. The same type of wet smear made with physiologic saline solution for the diagnosis of trichomoniasis can be used for non-specific vaginitis. Of special note is the marked absence of inflammatory white blood cells and acid-producing Döderlein's bacillus. Most helpful in making the diagnosis are the typical "clue cells," which are vaginal squamous epithelial cells covered by bacteria. They have a stippled appearance. Scanning electron microscopy has shown the bacteria clinging to the surface of the cells, not merely superimposed on them. If a drop of 10 percent potassium hydroxide is added to the discharge from H. vaginalis, a characteristic fishy odor is released. The alkaline substance causes release of the odorous amines, making possible this "whiff test." Culture of H. vaginalis is extremely difficult, requiring moist anaerobic conditions with immediate and careful plating on protease blood agar for 48 hours under 10 percent carbon dioxide. Since few physicians have this type of laboratory capability at hand, culture has been reserved for clinical research. H. vaginalis can also be recognized in the Papanicolaou smear that shows a background with myriads of small bacteria. These organisms are not cytotoxic and do not produce atypical changes in the squamous epithelial cells, as may Trichomonas vaginalis.

The treatment for H. vaginalis vaginitis, which had been the use of local sulfonamides, has now become rather controversial. H. vaginalis is usually resistant to sulfa in vitro. The Food and Drug Administration in 1980 found that "there is no adequate evidence that sulfanilamide and sulfisoxazol vaginal creams are effective in treating vaginitis caused by Candida albicans, Trichomonas vaginalis, and Haemophilus vaginalis."[15] Another recent study has shown an 80 percent cure rate using sulphonamide vaginal tablets,[12] but this could be due to reacidification of the vaginal pH. The usual treatment period for the sulfonamide vaginal creams and tablets (AVC, Sultrin, Vagitrol, Kori-Sulf, etc.) is once or twice daily for 1 to 3 weeks. Another recent study made the serendipitous discovery that metronidazole (Flagyl) 500 mg twice daily for 1 week was 98 percent effective in eliminating H. vaginalis vaginitis.[16]

Other oral antibiotics have also been used for treating H. vaginalis, with various success. Ampicillin is highly effective in vitro, but when given 500 mg 4 times a day for 5 to 7 days, is only 33 percent effective in treating H. vaginalis vaginitis in vivo. Tetracycline, which also appears effective in vitro, works poorly in vivo. Both antibiotics are frequently associated with overgrowth of Candida albicans. Cephalexin 500 mg, 4 times daily, has been used with fair results. Vaginal reacidification, with douches and buffered vaginal creams and jells, has also been effective and is used by many women who have chronic bacterial vaginitis to maintain an asymptomatic state. Since H. vaginalis vaginitis is a venereal disease, recurrences can be prevented only by simultaneous treatment of the sexual partner with metronidazole, or 5 days of ampicillin 500 mg 4 times daily, or tetracycline 250 mg 4 times daily. These schedules are not uniformly successful, and some investigators have also suggested 2 weeks of condom use or sexual abstinence for men to rid themselves of this infection. For women with reucrrent H. vaginalis vaginitis and extensive cervicitis, cervical cautery or cryosurgery is frequently helpful, by eliminating the excessive mucus production causing loss of vaginal acidity. Povidone-iodine (Betadine) vaginal douches and vaginal gel have been recommended for the treatment of non-specific vaginitis, but this regimen of therapy is difficult, prolonged, and likely to have poor patient compliance.

Vaginal bacterial cultures are frequently performed in an attempt to make a diagnosis of a specific bacterial pathogen, but proper interpretation depends on a knowledge of the normal vaginal flora. Many types of bacteria, including streptococci, staphylococci, E. coli, Hemophilus species, pseudomonas, proteus, Bacteroides, mycoplasma, and others, can be recovered from the vaginas of women without evidence of infection, as well as in those with vaginitis.[17] The vaginal flora depends on the patient's age, estrogen effect on the vaginal mucosa, and other factors influencing the balance of flora, such as recent antibiotic therapy or use of vaginal medications or douches. One should not attribute vaginitis to the presence of an unusual bacteria until the common causes of vaginitis (Candida, Trichomonas, and Haemophilus vaginalis) have been ruled out. Vaginal cultures in this situation may be helpful if the reporting laboratory can quantitate the bacteria, to allow the physician to identify the predominant organism. The patient must also have abstained for several days from douching or using any vaginal medications which contain bacteriocidal or bacteriostatic agents.

Stretococci are part of the normal vaginal flora, and rarely pathogenic in women during the reproductive years with normal amounts of vaginal estrogen and normal vaginal acidity. Patients with streptococcal vaginitis have a thin, purulent discharge, complain of burning and pruritus, and have severe vaginal inflammation. Streptococci may cause pelvic inflammatory disease in the postpartum or post-abortal period. Streptococcal vaginitis is best treated with vaginal estrogens when a deficiency exists, and with sulfonamide creams. Systemic antibiotics are reserved for the puerperal infections. Staphylococcal vaginitis is rare and usually associated with vulvar staphylococcal infections as well as with the administration of systemic antibiotics. The discharge is usually sticky and purulent, and the vaginitis resolves without special therapy with the resolution of the vulvar infection and discontinuation of antibiotics, allowing repopulation of the vagina by the lactobacilli. E. coli, which is frequently identified in normal vaginal flora, has been observed rarely as a vaginal pathogen. It produces a purulent, yellow-green exudate. This infection is usually caused by factors previously mentioned which alter the vaginal environment, and resolves without specific therapy.

ATROPHIC VULVOVAGINITIS

Atrophic vaginitis is the modern name for the condition formerly known as senile or senescent vaginitis. This change in name has made it easier for physicians to explain the problem to patients, since no woman wants to be told that her vagina is "senile." It is not a primary infection, but an inflammatory reaction, with ulceration and telangiectasia of the vaginal mucosa which has become thinned by inadequate estrogen. Atrophic vaginitis is seen following menopause in the late climacteric, or following castration by surgery or radiation. It occurs when the total endogenous estrogen production from ovaries, adrenal glands, and the extraglandular sites drops below a critical level which varies from one individual to another. Once this level has been reached, the vaginal epithelial cells no longer produce glycogen, and can no longer support lactic-acid-producing Döderlein bacilli. With the loss of vaginal acidity, there may be loss of resistance to pathogenic organisms, with secondary infection by *Candida albicans, T. vaginalis, H. vaginalis,* or other pathogenic bacteria.

Although atrophic changes occur at different rates in most women after menopause, the diagnosis of atrophic vaginitis should be reserved for those women who become symptomatic. Common irritative symptoms include dysuria, external burning, pruritus, tenderness, discharge, and dyspareunia. With the thinning of the vaginal mucosa, there is a decrease in elasticity, with shrinkage of the tissue, vaginal shortening, loss of rugal folds, and, when severe, the formation of intravaginal adhesions. The vaginal mucosa may be easily traumatized by intercourse or examination, causing spotting or bleeding from breaks in the vaginal mucosa. If this cannot be distinguished from uterine bleeding, a diagnostic currettage is necessary to exclude endometrial pathology. The type of discharge noted is highly variable, and may be purulent, serosanguinous, viscous, or watery, with color varying from gray to yellow. The acidity is always diminished with pH in the range of 5.5 to 7.5. Although many women complain of a vaginal discharge, others complain of vaginal dryness during intercourse from lack of lubrication. The urinary symptoms of frequency, urgency, dysuria, and nocturia may be related to atrophic changes of the estrogen-sensitive bladder trigone and urethra, without evidence of urinary tract infection. There may be eversion of the urethral mucosa at the meatus with the formation of a urethral caruncle. Vulvar changes usually occur after the vaginal changes and consist of thinning of the skin, with pruritus leading to excoriation and fissuring. The pubic hair becomes sparse and the labia minora regress in size with narrowing of the vaginal introitus. Dyspareunia may result from fissuring and ulceration of the vulvovaginal epithelium or stretching of the deeper inelastic tissues.

The diagnosis is usually apparent from the history: the patient's age, previous surgery, or radiation exposure. Again, the diagnosis is confirmed by a wet smear in saline which shows a background of many white blood cells and bacteria, and rules out trichomoniasis. In addition, the vaginal epithelial cells are of the parabasal and basal type, as would be expected with estrogen deficiency. The discharge should also be examined with potassium hydroxide to rule out candidiasis.

The obvious treatment for a condition of estrogen deficiency is of course estrogen replacement. This may be given either systemically or locally, depending on the severity and extent of the atrophic changes. If the patient has an atrophic vagina with no objective inflammatory symptoms, no treatment is necessary. If the patient's symptoms are only vaginal in nature, an estrogen vaginal cream will probably be sufficient. The most common creams are conjugated equine estrogens (Premarin cream, 0.625 mg/gm of cream), and dienestrol 0.01 percent (DV-Cream), using one-half applicator full intravaginally daily for 2 weeks. This allows relief of the symptoms and recornification of the vaginal epithelium. A well-cornified vaginal mucosa can then be maintained with the installation of the cream once or twice a week, depending on the patient's responses and needs. Systemic use of estrogens should be reserved for the young castrated patients and the menopausal patients with other systemic symptoms of estrogen deficiency, such as vasomotor instability (hot flashes) and atrophic urethrocystitis. The most common estrogen tablets are conjugated estrogens (Premarin): 0.3 gm, 0.625 mg, 1.25 mg, 2.5 mg; ethinyl estradiol (Estinyl): 0.02 mg and 0.05 mg; diethylstilbestrol: 0.1 mg, 0.05 mg, and 1.0 mg; and estradiol (Estrase): 1 mg and 2 mg tablets. The dosage chosen should be the minimum required to alleviate the patient's symptoms. These tablets should probably be given in a cyclic fashion (e.g., 3 weeks on and 1 week off). Within a few days after institution of estrogen therapy by either route, the vaginal epithelium thickens; the hemorrhagic spots, excoriations, and ulcerations disappear; normal flora and acidity return; and subjective symptoms are relieved. Persistent symptoms and signs of vaginitis following estrogen therapy should be re-investigated in the traditional fashion with wet smears of saline and potassium hydroxide, since restoration of vaginal glycogen and acid pH may allow secondary infection by Candida or potentiate an asymptomatic chronic Trichomonas infection. Contraindications to the use of estrogens include undiagnosed uterine bleeding, cancer of the breast, estrogen-dependent tumors, thrombophlebitis or a history of thrombophlebitis or thromboembolic disorders. Caution should be used in prescribing estrogens to patients with liver diseases, diabetes, hypertension, and fluid retention. For more complete prescribing information, the Physicians' Desk Reference [18] should be consulted. It should be remembered that when estrogens are given intravaginally, they are absorbed systemically, so that the contraindications are the same as with the oral tablets. Because of the recent association of prolonged estrogen use with a 5 to 15 times increased risk of developing endometrial cancer,[19] some patients are fearful of taking any estrogenic substances, and will chose to withstand a great deal of physical discomfort for their emotional well-being. In patients with atrophic vaginitis who are unable to use estrogens, an acid buffered vaginal jelly (Aci-Jel) can be used with limited success. This is probably most helpful in eliminating certain pathogenic bacteria. Atrophic vulvitis usually responds nicely to local corticosteriod creams such as hydrocortisone cream, 1 percent applied 4 times daily.

TREATMENT FOLLOW-UP

After completion of treatment for vaginitis, it is important to see the patient for follow-up examination. This is usually performed by the patient's private physician, depriving the emergency room physician, who made the diagnosis, the opportunity to evaluate the adequacy of his therapy. There may be reasons for persistent vaginitis after therapy other than recurrence of the original pathogens as discussed above.

Some physicians believe that treatment of Trichomonas vaginitis may cause Candida vaginitis, and treatment of Candida vaginitis may cause Trichomonas vaginitis. These empiric observations are likely to be based on the results of partial treatment of a mixed vaginal infection of trichomonads and Candida where only one pathogenic organism was discovered on initial evaluation. This emphasizes the importance of thorough examination of saline and potassium hydroxide wet smears; if both organisms are identified, specific agents should be used concomitantly to insure relief of the patient's symptoms. It has been suggested that povidone-iodine may be adequate therapy for this type of mixed infection.[20] *Trichomonas vaginalis* and *H. vaginalis* may co-exist in a mixed vaginal infection; metronidazole therapy is usually satisfactory in treating both of these pathogens.

Other patients with persistent or worse symptoms after treatment of vaginitis may in fact be exhibiting a reaction to the medication. For example, patients allergic to sulfa may develop a severe allergic vaginitis, with vaginal and vulvar erythema, edema, and pruritis, following the use of a sulfa vaginal cream. Examination of the vaginal discharge is usually negative for pathogens.

Lastly, the physician should be aware of the relatively rare entity of psychosomatic vulvovaginitis. This is seen in dependent and emotionally labile women with a long history of persistent vaginitis unsuccessfully treated by multiple physicians. There is usually a history of allergy to most vaginal preparations. Sexual inactivity is a direct result of the vaginitis, providing a secondary gain. Physical examination shows a lack of pathology on multiple occasions. Psychotherapy is often needed but the patients are usually reluctant to accept the suggestion of a psychophysiologic cause.[21]

REFERENCES

1. Gardner HL, Kaufman RH: Benign Diseases of the Vulva and Vagina. pp 149–229. C.V. Mosby, St Louis, 1969.
2. Hesseltine HC: Biologic and clinical import of vulvovaginal mycoses. Am J Obstet Gynecol 34:855, 1977.
3. Diddle, AW, et al: Oral contraception medications and vulvovaginal candidiasis. Obstet Gynecol 34:373, 1969.
4. Loh WP, and Baker GG: Fecal flora of men after oral administration of chlortetracycline or oxytetracycline. Arch Intern Med 95:74, 1955.
5. Syverson RE, et al: Cellular and humoral immune status in women with chronic Candida vaginitis. Am J Obstet Gynecol 134:624, 1979.
6. Davis JE, et al: Comparative evaluation of Monistat and Mycostatin in the treatment of vulvovaginal candidiasis. Obstet Gynecol 44:403, 1974.
7. Zuspan F: Management of patients with vaginal infections. J Reprod Med 9:1, 1972.
8. Kistner RW: Gynecology: Principles and Practice. 3rd Ed. Year Book Medical Publishers, Chicago, 1979.
9. Coutts WE, et al: Trichomonas vaginalis infection in the male. Br Med J 2:885, 1955.
10. Dykers Jr JR: Single-dose metronidazole for trichomoniasis: patient and consort. N Engl J Med 293:23, 1975.
11. Gardner HL, Dukes CD: Haemophilus vaginalis vaginitis: a newly defined specific infection previously classified "non-specific" vaginitis. Am J Obstet Gynecol 69:962, 1955.
12. Bhattacharyxa MN, Jones BM: Haemophilus vaginalis infection. J Reprod Med 24:71, 1980.
13. Gardner HL, Dukes CD: Haemophilus vaginalis vaginitis. Ann N Y Acad Sci 83:280, 1959.
14. Josey WE, et al: Corynebacterium vaginale (Haemophilus vaginalis) in women with leukorrhea. Am J Obstet Gynecol 126:574, 1976.
15. FDA Drug Bulletin: Vol 10, No 1, p 6, February, 1980.
16. Pheifer TA, et al: Non-specific vaginitis, role of Haemophilus vaginalis and treatment with metronidazole. N Engl J Med 289:1429, 1978.
17. Lavinson ME, et al: Quantitative bacteriology of the vaginal flora in vaginitis. Am J Obstet Gynecol 133:139, 1979.
18. Physician's Desk Reference. 34th Ed. Medical Economics, Oradell, NJ, 1980.
19. Smith DC, et al: Association of exogenous estrogen and endometrial carcinoma. N Engl J Med 293:1164, 1975.
20. Ratzan JJ: Monilial and trichomonal vaginitis-topical treatment with povidone-iodine preparations. Calif Med 110:24, 1969.
21. Dodson MG and Friedrich EG: Psychosomatic vulvovaginitis. Obstet Gynecol 51:235 No 1 Suppl, 1978.

10 Pediatric Gynecology

Gertrude J. Frishmuth

Emergencies in pediatric gynecology can be life-threatening as well as influential on the future reproductive capabilities of the child. It must be borne in mind, then, that the emergency room (ER) physician must assess the problem with the utmost competence and, if necessary, alert the gynecologist as soon as the patient is stabilized. Fortunately, however, the majority of pediatric gynecologic emergencies can be handled adequately by the ER physician, and the patient can be sent home, to be followed up later by either a pediatrician or a gynecologist.

EXAMINATION OF THE PATIENT

The position in which the patient is examined depends on the age and the size of the patient. The small child can be frog-legged in her mother's lap or in the supine position on the examination table. The premenarchal child may be able to use the stirrups. The knee-chest position is also recommended by some.[1] Regardless of the position used, it should be remembered that the examination is a stressful situation, and only when the physician is ready to proceed with the exam should the patient be placed properly. There is nothing more disconcerting to an 11 year old than to be placed in the dorsal lithotomy position, with feet in stirrups, and then have to wait for the physician to finish with another patient.

The type of genital examination performed will depend not only on the complaint but also on the age of the patient. It goes without saying that the external genitalia should be examined and particular attention paid to evidence of trauma, i.e., abrasions, lacerations, edema, ecchymoses. The location and extent of such evidence should be recorded. If a speculum examination is necessary and can be performed atraumatically, there are several recommended types. The small nasal speculum is appropriate for the small child. The

Huffman speculum with the blunted introducer is used for the premenarchal child.[2] A good light source is recommended. Recently the use of the veterinary otoscope specula with the standard otoscope head has shown great promise, giving excellent illumination for examination of the vagina.[3] It is unlikely that a narrow-bladed Pederson speculum could be used successfully in the pediatric patient.

A gynecologic examination may be of value when there is an abdominal mass, urinary complaints, or pain on defecation. A good abdominal examination is imperative and this should be done, if possible, in the supine as well as in the flexed-knee position. The small vagina of a child may not permit a bimanual pelvic examination, but a rectal or rectal-abdominal exam is usually easy to perform.

EMERGENCIES IN PEDIATRIC GYNECOLOGY

Trauma

History. The history of the circumstances surrounding the trauma is extremely important. To know how the trauma occurred will occasionally permit one to estimate the depth of the injury. Was there sharp or blunt injury and with what force, e.g., a thrown baseball bat, a fence-straddling, a fall on a bed post? Car accidents can produce a fractured pelvis with laceration or complete severance of the urethra. Sharp injuries give fresh hemorrhage and the site is evident. Although some edema may form, a hematoma is rare. Blunt trauma will lead to hematoma formation.[4] Occasionally the history reveals that the injury occurred several days or a week ago and only now is there active bleeding, due to sudden rupture of a concealed hematoma.

Physical. The physical exmaination should note all areas of trauma and the extent. An injury is defined as to size, location, and the amount of bleeding (if any), e.g., a 2 cm by 2 cm abrasion of the right labia majora with no active bleeding. It is wise to sketch on the admission form the perineum with the location of injuries, for documentation purposes. Ascertain, if possible, whether the patient can void or not, and note if there is frank hematuria. A speculum exam may be performed, and if there is no history of head trauma, small children may require sedation (e.g., chloral hydrate or phenobarbital). A rectal-abdominal exam is done to rule out an intraperitoneal injury (mass in the cul-de-sac) or a hematoma, especially of the vagina or recto-vaginal septum.

Differential Diagnosis. In the differential diagnosis of trauma in children, two unfortunate possibilities exist: suspicion of child abuse, and alleged rape. If the history is not too readily available, these are important considerations. The appropriate forms of the city or state should be filled out accurately and completely.

Treatment. If there is suspicion of a bladder or urethral injury, an intravenous pyelogram should be ordered. If intraperitoneal injury is a possibility, then a flat plate of the abdomen will help. The vulva is an extremely vascular area and has a rich anastamosis from branches of the external pudenal artery (off the femoral artery) and branches of the internal pudenal artery (a branch of the hypogastric artery). If there is active bleeding that can be controlled with cold compresses (ice packs), this is fortunate. Usually, however, the rich anastamosis does not permit control of vulvar hemorrhage by compression or ligation.[4] Ecchymoses and hematomas develop readily with blunt trauma. Superficial lacerations can be repaired after appropriate cleansing and prepping of the area. Sedation and local anesthesia are required. Chromic catgut (3-0), Vicryl, or Dexon suture material can be used. If, after repair, hematoma formation is occurring, it is necessary to take down the repair and look for bleeders. A pressure dressing should be applied after a repair, and if there is edema, ice packs are recommended. The pressure dressing is best done using perineal pads and a sanitary belt. The perineal pads are to be changed with each use of the bathroom. Since the perineum is a bacteria-laden area of the body, prophylactic antibiotics are suggested. In cases of alleged rape, most cities require a vaginal and/or cervical culture for gonorrhea. If it is impossible to stop the bleeding, then the patient must be taken to the operating room for general anesthesia, and the gynecologist or the surgeon notified. They should also be notified when there is any suspicion of a deep, penetrating injury. In these cases the patient must be taken to the operating room to rule out injury to the urethra, bladder, rectum, posterior fornix of the vagina, or intra- or retroperitoneal injury.

Follow-up. If there has been any surgical repair by the emergency room physician, that patient should be seen the next day. If the area looks good, then sitz baths with warm water 3 to 4 times a day for 10 to 15 minutes can be started, and continued for the next 3 or 4 days. Then the patient is seen again to check on the repair. The area is to be kept clean and dry. If the patient has lost a considerable amount of blood, she may have to be admitted overnight for observation and possible blood replacement. The gynecologist will follow the patient taken to the operating room.

Vaginal bleeding

History. In taking the history of vaginal bleeding, it is important to know if the bleeding occurred following trauma or was spontaneous. Was the bleeding preceded by a vaginal discharge? Is there any pain associated with the bleeding? The age of the patient is important. A history of maternal drug ingestion during the intrauterine life of the child is significant, since the youngest patient in whom clear cell adenocarcinoma developed was aged seven.[5] It is important to know if the child has had access to hormone preparations, specifically birth control pills.

Physical. The physical examination should include some reference to the developmental status of the child. Here the Tanner classification[6] of breast development and pubic hair is helpful. Menarche follows breast buds and pubic hair. The abdomen must be examined for masses, since pregnancy and ovarian tumors (notably granulosa cell) can produce vaginal bleeding. Examination of the external genitalia will help define the source of bleeding as genital, and not from the gastrointestinal tract or the urological system. Trauma (see above) can also be ruled out. A rectal examination in the emergency room may help rule out gross tumor or a foreign body in the vagina. A speculum examination should be done in all cases of vaginal bleeding. This may require general anesthesia and vaginoscopy by a gynecologist, depending on the age, history, and physical findings.

Differential Diagnosis. The differential diagnosis of vaginal bleeding in the pediatric patient includes: maternal diethylstilbestrol (DES) ingestion, ingestion of birth control pills by the patient, foreign bodies in the vagina (see below), tumors of the vulva,[2,7] uterovaginal sarcomas (sarcoma botyroides), precocious puberty (menses before age 9 with development of secondary sex characteristics), urethral prolapse, neonatal vaginal bleeding, menarche, trauma, severe vulvovaginitis (especially those secondary to streptococcal infections), conscious or unconscious scratching (e.g., masturbation or pruritis), pinworms, pregnancy, and, rarely, blood dyscrasias.

Treatment. Emergency room treatment of vaginal bleeding depends on the source and amount. Trauma (see above) is the leading cause of vaginal bleeding in children.[8] The next most common source is a foreign body in the vagina (see below). If the history indicates maternal drug ingestion (specifically DES), the child must be seen by a gynecologist for examination. Likewise, suspicion of neoplasms must be referred to a gynecologist. Urethral prolapse is best handled by a urologist or gynecologist, but immediate treatment, if there is bleeding, is cold compresses. Urethral prolapse can be mistaken for tumors at the introitus; therefore a search for a meatal opening and possible catheterization of the bladder may be necessary if obstruction is present. Neonatal vaginal bleeding is treated by benign neglect. It is secondary to estrogen withdrawal (maternal and placental) and will usually disappear within the first 2 weeks of life. It is necessary to consider pregnancy in the peri-menarchal child since incomplete abortion is seen in the 12 and 13 year old female. If a vulvovaginitis is suspected, then appropriate vaginal cultures (taken with a saline-soaked cotton swab) are taken. Severe vulvitis, secondary to scratching, can be treated with cold compresses. If moniliasis is documented, then treatment is instituted. Inflammatory vulvitis (e.g., neurodermatitis) can be treated with steroid cream.

Follow-up. Referral to a gynecologist for follow-up, regardless of the initial treatment, is essential. It is always necessary to rule out tumors in childhood as a cause of vaginal bleeding.

Abdominal Masses with Special Reference to Ovarian Tumors

History. In taking the history of a child with an abdominal mass, it is important to get the time relationship for the development of the mass. It can be discovered accidently by the parent while dressing the child, or increased girth may be noted by the child herself. Early diagnosis of abdominal tumors in children is difficult because the tumors are usually silent until they have assumed tremendous size.[9] A history of sudden, sharp pain that comes and goes may indicate torsion and untwisting of an adenexa. Analysis of age distribution shows that although ovarian neoplasms may occur at any age in childhood or adolescence, they tend to be most frequent at puberty, between the ages of 10 and 14.[10]

Physical. Abdominal examination should differentiate between solid and cystic masses by palpation and percussion. The genitalia should be examined carefully and a patent hymen should be noted. The valsalva maneuver by the patient will demonstrate an imperforate hymen as a bulging mass at the introitus. A transverse vaginal septum can be found on vaginal examination. A rectal-abdominal exam is valuable since in most cases an ovary in a child is not palpable. If it is palpable, it is abnormal.[10] A large mass with pressure and interference with venous return can result in edema of the lower extremities. Pain on walking can also be due to pressure from a large mass.

Differential Diagnosis. Approximately 50 percent of abdominal masses in children can be of a non-surgical nature (leukemias, lymphomas, Hodgkin's disease, etc.), and these must be ruled out.[11] Of the remaining that are surgical, approximately 50 percent are from the urinary tract. About 3 percent of malignancy in childhood and adolescence is related to the gynecologic system, and the ovarian tumor is the most frequent genital neoplasm found.[10] The differential diagnosis of an abdominal mass in addition to those mentioned above includes: pregnancy, hematocolpos and/or hematometra, massive ovarian edema,[12,13] appendiceal abscess, intussuseption, obstruction, and salpingo-oophoritis.

Treatment. The proper diagnosis may be made by taking a good history and doing a complete physical examination. The patient will usually have to be admitted for an abdominal mass (other than pregnancy) involving the gynecologic system. If torsion of an adenexa is entertained, immediate surgery may result in saving some normal ovarian tissue. Hemorrhage and infarction into an ovary may result in loss of that ovary. Since only 1 in 10 ovarian neoplasms are malignant, panic is not justified, but judicious concern is to be exercised.[10]

Follow-up. The patient with the diagnosis of an ovarian neoplasm or a mass involving the genital tract should be seen as soon as possible by a gynecologist. The future reproductive capabilities of the child can be influenced by the quick action of the emergency room physician.

Parasites

History. The actual complaint of the patient or the parent may lead to the diagnosis of a parasitic infestation. Nocturnal perianal itching or awakening during the night with burning and itching of the perineum is important evidence to elicit. Intense pruritus of the perineum which is aggravated by warmth and perspiration is significant. Of special interest is a history of recent exposure to fresh water swimming or sea bathing. If the patient has been sleeping with other family members, and/or has been exposed to contaminated fomites (toilet seats, clothing, and bed linen), this should be noted.

Physical. Inspection of the external genitalia is the most important part of the physical examination. Pinworm can be found around the anus, and on the perineum, and also have been seen filling the vagina. Crab lice, both louse and "nits," must be looked for carefully in the pubic hair. Any dermatitis of the vulva (with or without a concomitant body rash) and cutaneous burrows of the inguinal region and the genitalia should be noted.

Differential Diagnosis. Enterobius vermicularis (pinworm) is the most frequent cause of nocturnal perianal itching in children.[2,14] They can infest the vagina, and the patient may wake up in the middle of the night crying because of being bitten. The serpinginous cutaneous burrows of the Sarcoptes scabiei (scabies) can be found on the buttocks, the inguinal region, and the genitalia.[15] Phthirus pubis (crab lice) can be found in the pubic hair of the premenarchal child and give intense itching. Shistosome dermatitis ("swimmer's itch"), can involve the perineum as well as other body surfaces. It is the result of exposure to contaminated snails (either fresh water or marine). A prickling sensation is followed by skin wheals, then a rash with severe itching.[15]

Treatment. Pinworm is treated with mebendazole (Vermox), one chewable 100-mg tablet regardless of weight, or pyrvinium pamoate (Povan), 5 mg/kg orally as a single dose. The entire family should probably be treated, as reinfection can occur. Scabies is treated by the application of Kwell, a 1 percent lindane (hexachlorocyclohexane) ointment, after a hot soapy bath.[15] A second application is seldom necessary. Crab lice is treated with Kwell lotion, shampoo, or ointment. "Swimmer's itch" has no specific treatment, but antipruritic and antihistaminic lotions are of palliative value (e.g., calamine lotion).

Follow-up. The pediatrician should follow-up the parasitic infestations of children. The source of the infective agent may have to be found and, as mentioned above, the entire family may have to be treated to prevent reinfestation.

Foreign Body in the Vagina

History. The presence of a foul, unremitting discharge may indicate a foreign body in the vagina. If the discharge is also bloody, it usually means the foreign body has been present for 2 to 3 weeks. Any unusual sexual behavior or sexual assault in the history can be important. Occasionally, children have explained to them the birth process (because of a recent or imminent family addition), and they become oriented to the vaginal canal. They are naturally inquisitive and place something in the vagina. Pain on defecation may indicate a foreign body in the vagina.

Physical. On physical examination, the foul-smelling vaginal discharge may make the diagnosis. Cultures of the discharge should be taken. Occasionally the dark, black masses of rolled-up wads of toilet paper (the most common item), are visible at the introitus. Lavaging the vagina with warm water by gravity (using a 14F red rubber catheter attached to a 25 cc syringe) can remove loose pieces of debris. A speculum exam is necessary to assure complete removal of the object. Anesthesia may be required, depending on the age of the patient. If the foreign body is hard and embedded or is a sharp object, its removal may require anesthesia. A rectal examination may be all that is needed not only to make the diagnosis, but also to remove the item by stripping the vaginal canal. The knee-chest position of the child can be helpful in exposing the vaginal canal.

Differential Diagnosis. The differential diagnosis includes necrosing tumors of the vagina, vaginal infections (including gonorrhea), and pinworm.

Treatment. Removal of the foreign body is curative and should be followed by gentle lavage of the vagina with warm water. As noted above, anesthesia may be required. Betadine sitz baths may be necessary to clear the vault of the foul-smelling discharge even after removal of the foreign body. Appropriate antibiotics for positive cultures should be administered.[16]

Follow-up. The patient should be seen in 2 to 3 days to assure complete removal of the foreign body and cessation of the discharge. This can be done by the pediatrician. If there is a recurrence of the problem, there may be a need for a nurse or social worker to visit the home. Counseling may be necessary as the child may be trying desperately to gain attention. If there is any suspicion of child abuse, appropriate action should be taken.

CONCLUSION

Emergencies in pediatric gynecology are common, and for the most part can be handled effectively by the emergency room physician. Once the diagnosis is made and the physician realizes his limitations, the patient benefits by being seen appropriately. A rapport between the ER physician and the gynecologist can enhance the learning experience and at the same time give the patient the very best medical care.

REFERENCES

1. Emans SJ, Goldstein DP: The gynecologic examination of the prepubertal child with vulvovaginitis: use of the knee-chest position. Pediatrics 65:758–760, 1980.
2. Huffman JW: The Gynecology of Childhood and Adolescence. W.B. Saunders, Philadelphia, 1968.
3. Billmire ME, Farrell MK, Dine MS: A simplified procedure for pediatric vaginal examination: use of veterinary otoscope specula. Pediatrics 65:823–825, 1980.
4. Friedrich Jr EG: Vulvar Disease (Major Problems in Obstetrics and Gynecology, Vol. 9). W.B. Saunders, Philadelphia, 1976.
5. Herbst AL, Cole P, Colton T, et al: Age-incidence and risk of DES-related clear cell adenocarcinoma of the vagina and cervix. Am J Obstet Gynecol 128:43–50, 1977.
6. Tanner JM: Growth at Adolescence. 2nd Ed. Blackwell Scientific Publications, Oxford, 1962.

7. Tsontsoplides GC: Surgical management of extensive congenital hemangiofibrolipoma of the vulva in an infant. Am J Obstet Gynecol 136:260–261, 1980.
8. Esposito J: Current problems in pediatric gynecology. Resident & Staff Physician 132:23s–29s, 1977.
9. Gangai MP: Pediatric abdominal masses. Hospital Medicine pp 6–23, October 1978.
10. Barber HRK: Ovarian Carcinoma: Etiology, Diagnosis, and Treatment. Masson Publishing, New York, 1978.
11. Melicow MM, Uson AC: Palpable abdominal masses in infants and children: a report based on a review of 653 cases. J Urol 81:705–710, 1959.
12. Bangel WM: Massive ovarian edema. Female Patient pp 92–93, April 1978.
13. Kanbour AI, Salazar H, Tobon H: Massive ovarian edema. Arch Pathol Lab Med 103:42–45, 1979.
14. Emans SJH, Goldstein DP: Pediatric and Adolescent Gynecology. Little, Brown, Boston, 1977.
15. Brown HW: Basic Clinical Parasitology. Appleton-Century-Crofts, New York, 1969.
16. Rettig PJ, Nelson JD, Kusmiesz H: Spectromycin therapy for gonorrhea in prepubertal children. Am J Dis Child 134:359–363, 1980.

11 Bleeding During Pregnancy

William R. Crombleholme

Bleeding during pregnancy is always a worrisome event for both patient and physician. However, its significance in a given patient may range from an inconsequential episode to a life-threatening emergency. It is the aim of this chapter to outline the causes of bleeding during pregnancy and to provide guidelines for their assessment and management.

FIRST TRIMESTER

Spotting is one of the most common problems in the first trimester of pregnancy. Patients may complain that the blood seen is bright red, dark red, or even brown in color. To some extent the color of the blood may give a clue to its origin. Brownish colored spotting usually represents old blood which has been reduced by the acid Ph of the vagina over a period of time. Alternatively, bright red blood is usually associated with an acute bleed from a source outside the uterus. Not infrequently such spotting may be from the cervix as a result of the blunt trauma that may occur with normal intercourse.

The cervix, as all the other pelvic tissues, will undergo characteristic changes during pregnancy. One common alteration seen is that of eversion of the endocervical epithelium at the external os. This results from hyperplasia of the endocervical columnar epithelium in response to the hormonal changes associated with pregnancy. Such eversions are sometimes erroneously called "erosions," but they do not represent an inflammatory process at all. The exposed endocervical epithelium is friable and bleeds easily when a Pap smear is taken or after intercourse has occurred. In the latter circumstance, such spotting should not be assumed to be indicative of cervical neoplasia (although the two may certainly co-exist).

On speculum examination, the cervix will have an overall cyanotic tinge to it, and one or two red, raw, friable patches will be seen on the portio. For patients enrolled in prenatal care with a recent normal Pap smear, the bleeding points may be cauterized with silver nitrate and intercourse proscribed for 5 to 7 days to allow healing. If a Pap smear has not been obtained recently, it should be done at the time the patient is seen, before any cauterization of the cervix is performed.

Dark red spotting is usually indicative of uterine bleeding. This is not an infrequent occurrence in the first trimester of pregnancy. It may represent an isolated event, or presage an eventual spontaneous abortion. Such bleeding may, or may not, be accompanied by lower abdominal pain in the first half of pregnancy. When bleeding and cramping occur together, the cervical os is closed, and no tissue has been passed, the diagnosis of threatened abortion is made. Examination of the patient will reveal a tightly closed cervix. One may even see dark red blood oozing from the os. The only indicated therapy is bed rest and proscription of intercourse. Hormonal therapy has no place in the management of such patients. For those pregnancies which will proceed normally, hormonal therapy represents a needless teratogenic risk to the fetus. For those pregnancies which are destined to terminate, it only prolongs the time from the onset of symptoms until the final passage of tissue occurs.

When uterine bleeding, whether dark red or bright red, becomes heavy the possibility of a spontaneous abortion must be considered. Such abortions may be complete or incomplete. A complete abortion is when the products of conception are passed in their entirety. This is usually difficult to determine unless it fortuitously happens at the time of examination or the patient brings the passed tissue with her from home. In either event, inspection of the tissue will reveal an intact gestational sac with a clean, unbroken placental margin surrounding it.

More commonly, only a portion of the products of conception will have been passed. This is an incomplete abortion. The diagnosis is both descriptive and etiologic of the patient's bleeding. With separation of the placenta from its attachment to the endometrium, large maternal sinuses are ruptured. Cessation of blood flow into these sinuses occurs by contraction of the myometrium around the vessels supplying these sinuses. However, these contractions can occur only if the volume of the endometrial cavity has been reduced by the evacuation of the retained products of conception. On examination the vagina may be filled with blood and clots which should be manually removed. The cervix will be open and some tissue may be seen protruding through the os. If so, this tissue should be grasped with a ring forcep, or other suitable long blunt forcep, and gently removed. Not uncommonly, a significant bulk of tissue will be removed. This will allow the uterus to contract and help control the bleeding immediately. An intravenous infusion should be started with either normal saline or Ringer's solution, and pitocin should be added to the solution in a dose of 20 units per liter of fluid. Blood specimens should also be obtained for a complete blood count and crossmatching since in some patients the bleeding may be profuse enough to require transfusion. The patient, once stabilized, should undergo curettage as soon as possible because cessation of bleeding will occur only when the uterus has been completely emptied. Serious uterine infection and generalized sepsis as a result of prolonged retention of the products of conception will be avoided if a D&C is done soon after the diagnosis is made. Following the procedure, in the Rh negative, unsensitized patient, RH immune globulin should be administered to prevent sensitization. Mini-doses of 50 μg of Rh immune globulin is available for these cases.

The third major cause of bleeding in the first trimester is the bleeding associated with ectopic pregnancy. This topic is considered elsewhere so no further discussion need take place here.

SECOND TRIMESTER

Bleeding during the second trimester of pregnancy generally involves the same differential diagnoses as for first trimester bleeding, except an ectopic pregnancy is an extremely rare occurrence in the second trimester. However, since the pregnancy is more advanced with a larger placental site, the risk of significant hemorrhage with spontaneous incomplete abortions is proportionately increased. Nonetheless, the essential aspect of management remains evacuation of the uterus, which must be accomplished as quickly as is safely possible.

THIRD TRIMESTER

Bleeding during the third trimester of pregnancy truly spans the range of concern from normal physiologic "show" in association with the onset of labor, to life-threatening hemorrhage in association with placenta previa or abruptio placenta. As the latter two conditions represent true medical emergencies, it would perhaps be best to begin our considerations with these.

Placenta previa occurs when the placenta has implanted in the lower segment of the uterus and comes to lie over, or adjacent to, the internal os of the cervix. Depending on the extent of the latter relationship, four categories of placenta previa are described. Total placenta previa is when the internal os is completely covered by placenta. Partial placenta previa is when the internal os is partially covered by placenta. Marginal placenta previa is when the edge of the placenta is at the margin of the internal os. Lastly, a low-lying placenta is one whose implantation site is so close to the internal os that its edge can be palpated by digital examination through the cervix.

The type of placenta previa diagnosed will depend on the extent of cervical dilatation at the time of diagnosis, as well as the method of diagnosis. The diagnosis made by digital exam at the time of a "double set-up" (which will be discussed later) may be total if only a small amount of cervical dilatation has occurred; but might be partial, in the same patient, if examined at a later time when further dilatation has revealed the os to be only partially covered by placenta. Similarly, ultrasonic diagnoses of total or marginal placenta previa, earlier in pregnancy, may become marginal or low-lying when scanned later in pregnancy, after progressive growth of the uterus moves the placenta away from the area of the internal os.

While placenta previa can occur as a result of the chance implantation of the blastocyst in the lower segment of the uterus, certain conditions may predispose, or at least be found in association with, placenta previa. Multiparity and advancing maternal age seem associated with placenta previa, as does abnormal vascularization of the decidua resulting from inflammatory or atrophic changes. Alternatively, conditions resulting in large placentas, such as erythroblastosis or multiple fetuses, may also give rise to placenta previa as the growth of such placentas encroaches upon the area of the internal os. Overall, the incidence of placenta previa is about 0.5 percent of all pregnancies.[2]

The characteristic symptom of placenta previa is painless, bright red vaginal bleeding. The quantity of bleeding is significant, usually being at least equivalent to a cupful of blood, and frequently considerably more. Not uncommonly, the patient may be resting when the bleeding starts; the patient may awake at night to find herself in a pool of blood.

When patients in the third trimester of pregnancy come to the hospital with significant vaginal bleeding, they should be placed in a supine position with a slight degree of Trendelenburg. As the patient is recounting the events leading to her arrival at the hospital, the perineum should be visually inspected to determine if the bleeding has continued. This initial step will allow the physician to determine the urgency of the situation and consequently to establish a time frame for initial evaluation and management; i.e., stat or merely expeditiously. The maternal vital signs should be obtained. An intravenous infusion of normal saline or Ringer's lactate solution should be started. Blood obtained for hematocrit and hemoglobin, as well as for type and crossmatch for 2 to 4 units of whole blood, should be sent to the laboratory. While this is being accomplished, the essential aspects of the history can be obtained: the length of gestation based on the patient's last menstrual period and estimated date of confinement (EDC); the quantity of blood lost; the associated level and type of activity at the time of bleeding, and significant past obstetrical, medical, and surgical history.

Having completed the initial maternal evaluation, attention should then be turned to evaluation of the fetus. The presence of fetal heart tones should be ascertained as well as the fetal heart rate. The size of the uterus should be assessed by measuring the fundal height in centimeters from the top of the fundus to the upper edge of the symphysis pubis. This should roughly correspond to the gestational age estimated from the patient's EDC. The uterus should be evaluated with respect to tone, tenderness, and irritability. Bleeding because of placenta previa will be associated with a soft, non-tender, and non-irritable uterus. The position of the fetus should be determined by palpation to localize the head and the breech, and to learn whether or not the fetus has begun to enter the birth canal. This is useful information: with a placenta previa, the entrance to the birth canal, or inlet of the pelvis, will be occupied by the placenta. The fetus will be "floating" within the uterus and an empty space will be palpable abdominally above the pelvic brim and below the fetus.

Having thus established the status of both patients, mother and fetus, a definitive management plan can be formulated. Such a plan can be conservative or aggressive, depending upon the degree of maternal bleeding and the gestational age of the fetus. Most often the first episode of bleeding with placenta previa is self-limiting and of moderate degree. With that in mind, when a fetus is less than 36 weeks gestational age, the management plan is conservative: complete bed rest in the hospital, careful observation, no pelvic examinations, and confirmational evaluation of the diagnosis by ultrasound.

If a total placenta previa is found on ultrasound, the patient will require complete bed rest in the hospital until fetal pulmonary maturity can be confirmed by amniocentesis sometime after 36 weeks of gestation. At that time, delivery can be accomplished by cesarean section. If only a partial or marginal placenta previa or a low-lying placenta is found, the patient will require observation and bed rest in the hospital until no further bleeding is noted, generally a minimum of 5 to 7 days. Under those circumstances, if the patient lives relatively close to the hospital, has immediate and continuous access to rapid transportation to the hospital, and has a home setting which will permit complete bed rest, the patient may be discharged from the hospital with strict instructions to return at the first sign of any bleeding.

Alternatively, with a fetus of 36 weeks gestational age or more, or with continued heavy vaginal bleeding, irrespective of fetal gestational age, the management plan is decidedly aggressive. The first step is preparation for a "double set-up" examination. This examination is simply a pelvic examination performed in an operating room with the patient prepped and draped for cesarean section. A complete operative team—anesthesiologists, obstetricians, pediatricians, and nursing personnel—is present and ready to begin the operation if the vaginal examination confirms the diagnosis of placenta previa. The purpose of the double set-up examination is to permit differentiation between unusually heavy "show" associated with normal labor, placenta previa, and abruptio placentae, the second life-threatening cause of third trimester bleeding.

Abruptio placentae is simply the separation of the placenta, in part or entirely, from the normal implantation site in the uterus, prior to delivery of the fetus. As a consequence of this separation, open maternal sinuses continue to bleed so that blood, dark or bright red, dissects between the uterine wall and fetal membranes and appears in the vagina. Along with several other characteristics to be discussed later, vaginal bleeding with abruptio placentae differs from that with placenta previa in that it tends to be more profuse and is not self-limiting. In addition, in so-called "concealed" abruption, no external bleeding is seen at all. The blood accumulates in a huge clot behind the placenta. The overall incidence of abruptio placentae, when all degrees of premature separation of the placenta are included, approximates 0.5 percent. However, the incidence of separation extensive enough to cause fetal death is probably more on the order of 0.2 percent.[6]

The etiology of placental abruption remains obscure, although several factors seem associated and may be etiologic in its occurrence. Such varied factors as trauma, short umbilical cord, sudden decompression of the uterus, uterine anomalies or tumors, vena caval compression or occlusion, or even dietary deficiencies of folic acid have been invoked to explain the etiology of placental abruption with varying degrees of supportive evidence. Perhaps the most common and consistently found factor in association with placental abruption is maternal hypertension, either chronic or pregnancy-induced.

The clinical picture of a patient with placental abruption is considerably different from that of a patient with placenta previa. Unlike with previa, the patient usually notes associated pain with her vaginal bleeding, either periodic, from uterine contractions, or continuous. The continuous pain may be relatively localized to a particular part of the uterus, anteriorly or posteriorly. Both types of pain may even occur together. On examination, the uterus is tender to palpation. There is an increased basal tone. Contractions are easily stimulated by palpation. Fetal heart tones may be absent if the fetus has died, or, if present, may be normal, tachycardic, or bradycardic. The fetal position, when it can be ascertained by palpation through the tense uterine wall, is usually normal. The fetal head has often entered the birth canal as a result of the uterine contractions and labor.

Another important consideration in patients with placental abruption is the occurrence of consumptive coagulopathy. The incidence of this complication may vary. It has been reported in as many as 30 percent[6] of patients with abruptions severe enough to cause fetal death. The initiation of the coagulopathy in such cases results from the infusion of thromboplastin from the decidua and placenta into the maternal circulation. Such an additional complication, along with simple blood loss, both contained within the uterus behind the placenta and lost per vagina, can significantly influence the management of shock, often seen in patients with severe abruptions.

In placental abruption there is not the option of conservative management as in placenta previa. Only an aggressive approach is consistent with maternal survival and potential fetal salvage. On admission, after a brief maternal history is obtained relating to the acute events and the essential aspects of the patient's obstetrical and medical history, the maternal and fetal vital signs should be obtained. The presence or absence of fetal heart tones, and the rate if present, are essential. The maternal pulse and blood pressure are especially important since tachycardia and a "normal" blood pressure in a known hypertensive patient represent early signs of shock. An intravenous infusion of normal saline or Ringer's solution should be started immediately with a large gauge needle. If profuse vaginal bleeding is present, a central venous pressure catheter is advisable. As the intravenous catheter is inserted, blood should be collected for several important studies: hematocrit, hemoglobin, platelet count, fibrinogen, fibrin split-products, prothrombin time (PT), partial thromboplastin time (PTT), electrolytes, blood urea nitrogen (BUN), creatinine, and a sample for typing and crossmatching for at least 4 units of fresh whole blood.

If signs of maternal shock are already present, the crystalloid infusions of saline or Ringer's solution should be supplemented with colloids, such as albumin, until whole blood can be obtained for transfusion. In the presence of signs of shock, if the coagulation profile, including platelet count, fibrinogen, PT and PTT, is normal, a central venous pressure line should be introduced via either the internal jugular vein, the subclavian vein, or a long line from an antecubital vein. The importance of a normal coagulation profile before placing a central line cannot be overemphasized. An initial assessment of the patient's coagulation status can be gained simply from observation of clot formation in the tubes of blood collected at the start of the intravenous infusion. Subsequently, first the platelet count, followed by the fibrinogen level and then the PT and PTT, will complete the picture of the patient's coagulation status. Since a central venous line necessarily involves puncture of a large deep-seated vein, such attempts in the presence of a coagulopathy could result in compressive hematomas of the neck or in hemothorax. As a complement to the central venous pressure line, the placement of a Foley catheter in the bladder will allow accurate and timed recordings of urinary output. The problem of renal failure in patients with abruptio placenta is largely a matter of renal hypoperfusion due to hypovolemia. The central line will allow the safe administration of the large amounts of blood and fluids often needed in these patients. Maintenance of good urinary output will reflect the successful correction of these deficits.

With completion of the assessment of maternal status and initiation of corrective measures to combat shock if present, attention must then be turned to delivery. In this context, an understanding of two aspects of fetal status is essential. First, fetal gestational age has no bearing on the management of abruptio placenta. Secondly, the mode of delivery will in large measure be determined by whether or not the fetus is alive.

With a live fetus, the only hope for fetal salvage is by expeditious delivery. This usually means cesarean section. Prior to surgery, however, the patient must be examined vaginally, since on occasion, enough time will have elapsed from the onset of symptoms for the uterine contractions stimulated by the abruption to have effected complete dilatation and effacement. The fetus can then be delivered vaginally. With a dead fetus, the mode of delivery is dictated by maternal indications.

When the patient is in labor and progressing well in dilatation and effacement, a vaginal delivery should be planned after the patient's hemodynamic status is stabilized. If the patient is not in labor but has signs of a total abruption, a dead fetus, and signs of shock with or without consumptive coagulopathy, management must be individualized. In these patients, stabilization with fluid and blood replacement is possible. Labor is induced with oxytocin and vaginal delivery effected in a reasonable period of time. In other patients, particularly those with severe consumptive coagulopathy, it may become necessary to evacuate the uterus surgically. This will stop the continued bleeding into the uterine cavity and prevent the continuation of the coagulopathy by preventing further thromboplastin release. In such situations one may even need to "feed the fire" for a brief period of time by administration of cryoprecipitate or fresh frozen plasma and possibly even platelets. This is usually necessary only prior to the operative procedure itself, since after delivery these patients improve very rapidly. A relatively stable status is attained within 6 to 8 hours of delivery. An almost normal coagulation profile is present 24 hours after delivery.

Having considered the catastrophic causes of third trimester bleeding, one must lastly consider a "normal" cause of bleeding in the third trimester, that associated with the onset of normal labor. The result of uterine contractions in labor is to effect effacement and dilatation of the cervix. During the latter process, there is often rupture of small blood vessels in the endocervix. In these circumstances, the blood is usually dark red and is most often mixed with mucous and, therefore, quite viscous. This type of bleeding can be confirmed historically since the patient will be at, or close to, her expected date of confinement, will note the onset of regular uterine contractions at progressively decreasing time intervals, and will usually have noted the appearance of the blood sometime after the contractions have started. After the appropriate history and abdominal examination have eliminated the possibilities of placenta previa or abruption, a simple vaginal examination will confirm the diagnosis of a "bloody show" in a patient in labor.

Since patients view the cessation of cyclic vaginal bleeding as the hallmark of a normal pregnancy, the occurrence of an episode of vaginal bleeding during pregnancy is at least a troubling, if not frightening, experience for the patient. Her anxiety, whether appropriate or exaggerated, may color her description of her symptoms and may significantly influence her interactions with her physician. For this reason, it is essential that physicians who care for such patients maintain an awareness of the spectrum of problems that bleeding during pregnancy may represent. A thorough and detailed history of events surrounding the bleeding episode, along with careful evaluation of the abdomen, will often establish the diagnosis and avoid the error of an inappropriate pelvic exam. At the same time, those instances where pelvic examination is both warranted and necessary will be identified and appropriate preparations will have been made. In this way the appropriate care of both mother and fetus will be assured.

REFERENCES

1. Bowie JD, Rochester D, Cadkin AV, et al: Accuracy of placental localization by ultrasound. Radiology 128:177, 1978.
2. Brenner WC, Edelman DA, Hendricks CH: Characteristics of patients with placenta previa and results of expectant management. Am J Obstet Gynecol 132:180, 1978.
3. Crenshaw Jr C, Jones DED, Parker R: Placenta previa: a survey of 20 years experience with improved perinatal survival by expectant therapy and cesarean delivery. Obstet Gynecol Surv 28:461, 1973.
4. Hibbard BM, Jeffcoate RNA: Abruptio placentae. Obstet Gynecol 27:155, 1966.
5. Knab DR: Abruptio placentae. Obstet Gynecol 52:625, 1978.

6. Pritchard J, Brekken A: Clinical and laboratory studies on severe abruptio placentae. Am J Obstet Gynecol 97:681, 1967.
7. Pritchard JA, Mason R, Corley M, Pritchard S: Genesis of severe placental abruption. Am J Obstet Gynecol 108:22, 1970.
8. Pritchard J, MacDonald P, Eds: Williams Obstetrics. 16th Ed. Appleton-Century-Crofts, New York, 1980.

Index

Page numbers followed by f represent figures; page numbers followed by t represent tables.

Abdomen
  acute
    appendicitis as, 31–32
    cholecystitis as, 34
    concurrent pregnancy and, 30t
    degenerating fibroid as, 33–34
    ovarian cysts as, 33
    pancreatitis as, 34–35
    pregnancy and, 25–37
    renal or ureteral stones as, 33
    urinary tract infection as, 32
  general examination of, 6
  gunshot wound of, 35
  lower, pain in, 61–79. *See also* Lower abdominal pain.
  masses of, pediatric, 130–131
  painful, general evaluation of, 30
Abortion
  alcohol consumption and, 16
  anesthetic gases and, 17
  complete, 136
  early first trimester, 16–17
  first trimester
    ectopic pregnancy and, 65
    pelvic inflammatory disease and, 73
  incomplete, 136–137
Abruptio placentae, 139–142
  central venous pressure line in, 141
  clinical picture in, 140
  coagulation status in, 141
  concealed, 139
  consumptive coagulopathy in, 140
  fetal considerations in, 141
  history and examination in, 140–141
  incidence of, 139–140
  vaginal delivery in, 141
Acute abdomen. *See* Abdomen, acute.
Adenitis, mesenteric, 77
Adenoma, hepatocellular, 106
Adnexa, examination of, 8
Age
  gestational, teratogenesis of drugs and, 14–17, 15f
  patient, 2
Alcohol consumption and abortion, 16
Amenorrhea, post-pill, 106
Analgesics and pregnancy, 19
Anemia, microangiopathic hemolytic, 43
Anesthetic gas exposure and abortion, 17
Antibiotics
  candidiasis and, 114–115
  pregnancy and, 18
Anticoagulants in pregnancy, 19
Anticonvulsants in pregnancy, 19–20
Antihistamines in pregnancy, 21–22
Antinauseants in pregnancy, 21–22
Appendicitis, 76–77
  children and, 77
  pelvic inflammatory disease vs, 76–77
  pregnancy and, 31–32
    diagnosis of, 31–32
    incidence of, 31
    premature labor and, 31
  symptoms of, 76
Asthma in pregnancy, 56–57
  evaluation of, 56
  therapy for, 56–57, 57t

Bendectin, 22
Birth control pill. *See* Oral contraceptive.
Bleeding, vaginal. *See* Vaginal bleeding.
Blood volume in preeclampsia, 43
Bloody show, 142
Breast examination, 6
Braxton-Hicks contractions, 28

Cancer
  chemotherapy for, candidiasis and, 115
  oral contraceptives and, 107
Candidiasis vaginitis, 113–116
Cardiovascular system in pregnancy, 28–29, 54
Cervix
  early pregnancy and, 135–136
  examination of, 8
  intrauterine contraceptive devices and, 110
Chadwick's sign, 27
Child(ren). *See* also Pediatric gynecology.
  appendicitis in, 77
  lower abdominal pain in, 61–62. 62t
  pelvic examination of, 9, 127–128
  sexual assault of, 82
  vaginal bleeding in, 82–84, 82t
Chemotherapy, 16
Cholecystitis in pregnancy, 34
Clomiphene citrate and teratogenesis, 16
Congenital malformation, 12

Consumptive coagulopathy, 140
Contraception
  effectiveness of, 103
  patient history of, 3
  types of, 103–104
Contraceptive problems, 103–112. *See also various contraceptives.*
Contractions, Braxton-Hicks, 28
Coronary disease and oral contraceptives, 107
Corticosteroids in pregnancy, 20
Crab lice, 132
Culdocentesis
  ectopic pregnancy and, 68
  pelvic inflammatory disease and, 73
Curretage in vaginal bleeding, 88
Cyst
  ovarian, pregnancy and, 33
  paraovarian, tubal torsion and, 75–76

Diabetic ketoacidosis in pregnancy, 50–53
  clinical studies in, 51
  fetal viability and, 53
  fluid and electrolyte abnormalities in, 52
  insulin therapy in, 51–52
  pathophysiologic changes in, 51
  phosphate depletion in, 52–53
  potassium loss in, 52
  precipitating causes of, 51t
  relative or absolute insulin deficiency in, 51
  treatment of, 53t
Diabetes mellitus and candidiasis, 114
Diethylstilbestrol, 20
Disseminated intravascular coagulation, 44
Diverticula of sigmoid colon, 77
Döderlein's bacillus, 113
Drugs in pregnancy, 11–23. *See also* Teratogenesis.
  analgesics, 19
  antibiotics, 18
  anticoagulants, 19
  anticonvulsants, 19–20
  antihistamines and antinauseants, 21–22
  Bendectin, 22
  corticosteroids, 20
  diethylstilbestrol, 20
  embryotoxic, 18t
  evaluation of, 12–14
    animal models in, 12
    case reports in, 13–14
    epidemiologic studies in, 13
  frequency of exposure to, 12
  hormones, 20–21
  lithium, 21
  psychotropic, 21
  teratogenic potential of, 14–17, 15f, 18t
    clomiphene citrate and, 16
    first 2 weeks of gestation and, 16
    genetic constitution and, 14
    gestational age and, 14–17, 15f
    late pregnancy and labor and, 17
    LSD and, 16
    male factor in, 16
    placental transfer in, 14
    weeks 3 to 7 of gestation and, 17
    week 12 to term and, 17
  testosterone, 20–21

Eclampsia, 40–42
  antihypertensive therapy for, 41
  clinical symptoms of, 40
  delivery in, 42
  mortality incidence in, 39
  protection of mother in, 41
  sedative anticonvulsants in, 41
  treatment of, 40, 41t
  urinary output in, 41–42
Ectopic pregnancy, 64–69, 63t
  abdominal pain and vaginal bleeding in, 66
  abdominal and pelvic tenderness in, 67
  blood values in, 67
  body temperature in, 66
  classic history in, 65–66
  culdocentesis in, 68
  early pregnancy complications with symptoms similar to, 69–70
  fertility after, 64
  first trimester abortion and, 65
  intra-abdominal bleeding with, 64
  intrauterine contraceptive device and, 65, 109–110
  laparoscopy in, 68–69
  mortality rate with, 64
  pelvic inflammatory disease in, 64–65
  pregnancy testing in, 67
  previous tubal sterilization and, 65
  progesterone-only birth control pill and, 65
  ruptured, 70–71
    emergency room management of, 70–71
    increasing vascular volume in, 71
    orthostatic hypotension and, 70–71
  shock in, 66
  symptoms of, 63t
  tubal disease in, 65
  ultrasound imaging in, 67
  vaginal bleeding in, 95
Embolism, pulmonary, pregnancy and, 57–58
Endometriosis, 76
Enteritis, regional, 77
Epidemiologic studies of teratogenicity, 13
Examination, 6–9
  general, 6–7
    abdomen in, 6–7
    breasts in, 6
    uterus in, 6
  pelvic, 79, 7t

Fallopian tube torsion, 75–76
Fetal hydantoin syndrome, 19–20
Fetus
  abruptio placentae and, 141
  diabetic ketoacidosis and, 53
  masculinization of, 21
  placenta previa and, 138–139
Fibroid, degenerating, pregnancy and, 33–34

Gametogenesis and drug effects, 14–16
Gastrointestinal system in pregnancy, 29
Genetics, fetal, teratogenesis and, 14
Gonorrhea, 71
Gunshot wound of abdomen, 35

Heart disease in pregnancy, 54
Hegar's sign, 27
Hepatocellular adenoma, 106
Hirsutism, 91
History, 2–6, 2t
  bleeding in, 5
  data base in, 2–3
    age of patient, 2
    contraceptive methods, 3
    menstrual history, 3
    parity of patient, 2–3
    sexual activity, 3
  pain in, 3–5
    menstruation and, 4
    site and radiation of, 3–4
    systemic upset and, 4–5
    vaginal discharge and, 4
  trauma in, 6
  vaginal discharge in, 5–6
Hormone therapy in pregnancy, 19–20
Hydrosalpinx and tubal torsion, 75–76
Hyperandrogenism, 90–94
  female, 86
  laboratory testing in, 90
  pregnancy testing in, 93–94
  site of overproduction in, 92–93
  symptoms of, 90
  treatment of
    acne and hirsutism, 91
    failure of, 93
    ovarian suppression in, 92
    pregnancy and, 90–91
    progestational agent or birth control pills in, 93
Hypermenorrhea, 94
Hypertension
  chronic
    superimposed preeclampsia and, 42–45. *See also* Preeclampsia.
    without superimposed preeclampsia, 45–46
  oral contraceptives and, 106
  pregnancy and, 39–47. *See also* Eclampsia; Preeclampsia.
  pregnancy-induced, 42–45
Hypotension, orthostatic, ectopic pregnancy and, 70–71

Intracranial vascular catastrophes, 105–106
Intrauterine contraceptive devices, 107–110
  bleeding with, 109
  cervical changes with, 110
  complications with, 107t
  ectopic pregnancy with, 65, 109–110
  expulsion of, 107–108
  infection with, 110
  pelvic pain with, 63
  perforation with, 108–109
  pregnancy with, 103–104, 109
Intussusception, 77

Ketosis, starvation, 50

Labor, premature, appendicitis and, 31
Laparoscopy in ectopic pregnancy, 68–69
Lithium in pregnancy, 21
Lower abdominal pain, 61–79
  appendicitis and, 76–77
  ectopic pregnancy, 64–69, 63t
  endometriosis and, 76
  first trimester pregnancy and, 62–63
  IUD and, 63
  ovarian or Fallopian tube torsion in, 75–76
  pediatric age group with, 61–62, 62t
  pelvic inflammatory disease, 71–75
  postmenopausal age group with, 63, 63t
  reproductive age group with, 62–63, 62t
LSD, 16

Male and teratogenesis, 16
Menarche, 61
  early anovulatory periods after, 84–85
Menorrhagia, 94
Menstruation
  abnormal bleeding and, 5
  history of, 3
  pain in, 4
  pregnancy prior to, 26–27
Microangiopathic hemolytic anemia, 43
Musculoskeletal system in pregnancy, 30
Myomas, uterine, pregnancy and, 33–34

Obstetrics. *See* Pregnancy.
Oral contraceptives, 104–107
  candidiasis and, 114
  complications of, 104t
    major, 105–107
      coronary disease and cancer as, 107
      hepatocellular adenoma as, 106
      hypertension as, 106
      post-pill amenorrhea as, 106
      thromboembolic and intracranial disease, 105–106
    minor, 105
  effectiveness of, 104
  progesterone-only, ectopic pregnancy and, 65
Ovary
  cysts of, pregnancy and, 33
  torsion of, 75–76
  tumors of, child with, 82, 130–131

Pancreatitis in pregnancy, 34–35
Parasites, 131–132
Pearl formula, 103
Pediatric gynecology, 127–134. *See also* Child(ren).
  abdominal masses and ovarian tumors in, 130–131
    differential diagnosis in, 131

Pediatric gynecology (cont.)
follow-up in, 131
history in, 130–131
physical examination in, 131
treatment of, 131
emergencies in, 128–133
parasites in, 131–132
differential diagnosis in, 132
follow-up in, 132
history in, 131–132
physical examination in, 132
treatment in, 132
patient examination in, 127–128
trauma and, 128–129
differential diagnosis in, 128
follow-up in, 129
history in, 128
physical examination in 128
treatment in, 128–129
vaginal bleeding and, 129–130
differential diagnosis in, 130
follow-up in, 130
history in, 129
physical examination in, 129–130
treatment of, 130
vaginal foreign body in, 132–133
differential diagnosis in, 133
follow-up in, 133
history in, 132
physical examination in, 132–133
treatment in, 133
Pelvic examination, 7–9, 7t
adnexa in, 8
bimanual, 8
cervix in, 8
patient relaxation and, 7
pouch of Douglas in, 9
rape and, 9
source of bleeding and, 8
systematic approach in, 7
uterus in, 8
vagina in, 7
vulva in, 7
young girl and, 9, 127–128
Pelvic inflammatory disease, 71–75. *See also* Salpingitis.
antibiotic therapy in, 74
appendicitis vs, 76–77
bacterial culture in, 73
blood values in, 73
culdocentesis in, 73
ectopic pregnancy and, 64–65
first trimester abortion and, 73
laparoscopy in, 73–74
outpatient treatment of, 74, 74t
visual diagnosis of, 72
Pinworm, 132
Placenta previa, 137–139
categories of, 137
diagnosis of, 137–138
double set-up examination in, 139
examination and history in, 138
fetal evaluation in, 138–139
incidence of, 138
management of, 139
predisposing conditions in, 138
symptoms of, 138
Placental transfer of drugs, 14
Postmenopausal age group, lower abdominal pain in, 63, 63t
Pouch of Douglas, 9
Preeclampsia, 42–45
blood loss in, 43
blood volume in, 43
coagulation mechanism in, 43
disseminated intravascular coagulation in, 44
drug treatment of, fetal effects of, 44
microangiopathic hemolytic anemia in, 43
treatment of, 44–45
volume overload in, 43
Pregnancy
abnormal vaginal bleeding in, 85–86
acute abdomen in, 25–37, 30t
acute medical emergencies in, 49–59
asthma in, 56–57
candidiasis in, 114
cardiovascular system in, 54
diabetic ketoacidosis in, 50–53
diagnosis of, 26–27
drugs in, 11–23
ectopic, 64–69, 63t. *See also* Ectopic pregnancy.
emergency room signs and symptoms of, 26t
first trimester
bleeding in, 135–137
cervix in, 135–136
complete abortion and, 136
incomplete abortion and, 136–137
lower abdominal pain in, 62–63
spotting in, 135
symptoms similar to ectopia in, 69–70
uterine bleeding in, 136
heart disease in, 54
hypertensive disorders of, 39–47. *See also* Eclampsia; Preeclampsia.
intrauterine contraceptive devices and, 109
physiologic changes during, 27–30
cardiovascular changes as, 28–29
gastrointestinal changes as, 29
musculoskeletal changes as, 30
reproductive tract anatomy as, 28
reproductive tract function as, 28
respiratory changes as, 29
urinary changes as, 29
prior to menstruation, 26–27
pulmonary edema in, 54–56
pulmonary embolism in, 57–58
second trimester, bleeding in, 137
third trimester
abruptio placentae in, 139–142
bleeding in, 137–142

bloody show in, 142
placenta previa and, 137–139
trauma during, 35–36
vaginal bleeding during, 26
Psychotropic drugs and pregnancy, 21
Puberty, precocious, 83–84
pseudoisosexual, 84
true form, 83–84
Pulmonary edema in pregnancy, 54–56
cardiac surgery for, 55–56
fetal well-being and, 55
monitoring in, 55
onset of, 54–55
treatment of, 55
Pulmonary embolism in pregnancy, 57–58
Pyelonephritis during pregnancy, 32

Rape
child and, 82
pelvic examination in, 9
Renal stones during pregnancy, 33
Reproductive age group
lower abdominal pain in, 62–63, 62t
vaginal bleeding in, 84–95
Reproductive tract in pregnancy
anatomy of, 28
function of, 28
Respiratory system in pregnancy, 29

Salpingitis, 71–75. *See also* Pelvic inflammatory disease.
classic history in, 72
frequency of symptoms in, 72
Scabies, 132
Sexual activity, 3
Sexual assault. *See* Rape.
Sigmoid colon diverticula, 77
Spermatogenesis and drug effects, 14–16
Starvation ketosis, 50
Streptococcal vaginitis, 121–122
Swimmer's itch, 132

Teratogen, soft, 13
Teratogenesis. *See also* Drugs in pregnancy.
criteria for drug in, 14
drug potential in, 14–17, 15f, 18t
epidemiologic studies of, 13
laboratory animals and, 12–13
male mediated, 16
Testosterone and pregnancy, 20–21
Thromboembolic disease with oral contraceptives, 105
Trauma
history of, 6
pediatric gynecology and, 128–129
pregnancy and, 35–36
Trichomoniasis, 117–119
Tridione syndrome, 20
Tubal sterilization and ectopic pregnancy, 65
Tumors, ovarian, pediatric, 82, 130–131

Ultrasound imaging in ectopic pregnancy, 67
Ureteral stones during pregnancy, 33
Urinary system in pregnancy, 29, 32
Uterine bleeding in early pregnancy, 136
Uterus
general examination of, 6
palpation of, 8

Vagina
inspection of, 7
pediatric, foreign body in, 132–133
Vaginal bleeding
abnormal, 81–101
anovulatory, 86–90
continuous estrogen stimulation in, 87
curretage in, 88
minor, 87–88
older patient with, 87
parenteral hormonal therapy in, 88–90
treatment of, 89t
young patients with, 87
history of, 5
intermenstrual, 5
intrauterine contraceptive device and, 109
massive, 94
mid-cycle, 94
older patient with, 95–98, 96t
anatomic problems in, 95
cancer incidence in, 96
estrogen administration in, 96
post-menopausal bleeding in, 96
progesterone administration in, 97–98
tissue sampling in, 96–97
pediatric, 129–130
post-menopausal, 96
pregnancy and, 26, 135–143
premenstrual, 94
reproductive age group with, 84–95
anatomic defects in, 86
anovulatory bleeding in, 86–90
coagulation defects in, 86
ectopic pregnancy in, 95
endocrine system abnormalities in, 86
etiologies of, 85–86, 86t
hyperandrogenism in, 86, 90–94
laboratory tests in, 86
mid-cycle bleeding in, 94
pregnancy complications in, 85
pre-menstrual staining in, 94
young, 85
source of, 8
unresponsive, 98–99
hypogastric artery ligation in, 98–99
surgical control of, 98
transcatheter embolization in, 99
very young patient and, 82–84, 82t
bacterial infections in, 83
causes of, 82
monilial vaginitis in, 82–83
ovarian tumors in, 82
pelvic examination in, 82

Vaginal bleeding (cont.)
precocious puberty in, 83–84
sexual assault or trauma in, 82
Vaginal discharge
history of, 5–6
pain and, 4
type of, 7
Vaginitis, 113–125
atrophic, 122–124
cause of, 122
diagnosis of, 123
symptoms of, 122
treatment of, 123–124
Candida, 113–116
antibiotics and, 114–115
cancer chemotherapy and, 115
diabetes mellitus and, 114
diagnosis of, 115
oral contraceptives and, 114
pregnancy and, 114
recurrent, 116
symptoms of, 114, 114t
treatment of, 115–116, 116t
vaginal glycogen in, 114
diagnostic factors in, 114t
monilial, child with, 82–83
non-specific bacterial, 119–122
bacteria in, 119
bacterial cultures in, 121
diagnosis of, 120
predisposing factors in, 120
spread of, 120
streptococci in, 121–122
symptoms in, 119–120
treatment of, 120–121
streptococcal, 121–122
treatment follow-up in, 124
Trichomonas, 117–119
asymptomatic, 117
chronic, 117
diagnosis of, 118
predisposing factors in, 118
sexual contact in, 117
spread of, 117–118
symptoms of, 117
treatment of, 118–119
Vulva, inspection of, 7
Vulvovaginitis. *See* Vaginitis.